WILD MEDICINE
Summer

Other books in the series

WILD MEDICINE

Summer

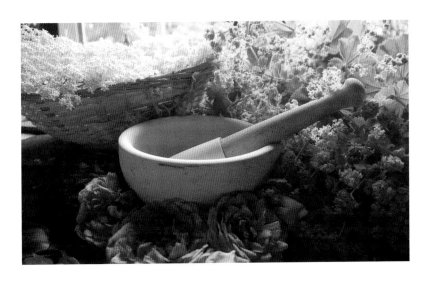

Ali English

Aeon Books

Disclaimer

The intent of this book is solely informational and educational. The information and suggestions in this book are not intended to replace the advice or treatments given by health professionals. The author and publisher have made every effort to present accurate information. However, they shall be neither responsible nor liable for any problem that may arise from information in this book.

First published in 2019 by
Aeon Books Ltd
12 New College Parade
Finchley Road
London NW3 5EP

British Library Cataloguing in Publication Data

A C.I.P. for this book is available from the British Library

ISBN: 978–1–91159–767–4

Printed in Great Britain by Bell & Bain Ltd, Glasgow

www.aeonbooks.co.uk

Contents

Summer

About the Author

Herbalist Ali English has been passionate about herbs from a young age and went on to study herbal medicine at Lincoln University, graduating in 2010 with a BSc (Hons). Since then, she has set up a practice in Lincolnshire that focuses on offering herb walks, workshops and a variety of related services, in which she tries to convey her love of our native herbs and wildflowers to anyone who will listen. *Wild Medicine: Summer* is her first book, with many more to follow.

Acknowledgements

For Matt, for his constant unswerving support and love, and for his patience with my ongoing plant obsession. Here's to many, many more years together, my Viking!

For Dafydd, for boots up the backside when I need them, and for sending this opportunity my way in the first place.

For my workshop attendees, and those who have come to my various herb talks and walks – thank you for the constant belief, encouragement and enthusiasm which continuously encourages me to keep learning and growing.

And for my family – who have put up with my babbling about plants for a very long time now, and generally without too many martyred expressions of patience!

Thank you all – I am where I am now because of you all, and I'm beyond grateful.

Preface

Welcome to *Wild Medicine: Summer*. It is my hope that this series of seasonal books will provide a source of information and kindle a keen delight in the glories of our native plants, both those growing in the hedgerows and those weedy adventurers tucked into nooks and crannies in our own gardens.

Plants have long been a passion of mine, ever since a bespectacled girl child of 13 asked for a garden and was given a small, round plot with four herbs and a sundial in it, plus a copy of *Culpeper's Herbal*. Three years later, that small plot boasted more than 40 herbs, and I was badgering my mother for more space.

The obsession went on from there, and many years later I graduated from university and began building myself a career working with the plants that have delighted, inspired and enchanted me for so long. It is difficult to ever feel alone in the world if you cultivate a friendship with the local wild plants – everywhere you look, you will see them eking out a living for themselves, from the wily and determined dandelion tucking itself into cracks between paving slabs, to the tall, elegant willow and balsam poplar by the river in my home city of Lincoln, hawthorn in hedgerows and poppies in brilliant red swathes across farmland in late summer. Plants are all around us, and over time they have become a true need for me, like water and food, air and freedom. Indeed, they are deeply entwined in my very blood and body, as they are for all of us – we inhale as they exhale, and we exchange breaths with plants constantly, sharing the same air.

It is my aim that these books will provide hedgerow travel books to tuck into a pocket and take along with you in the warmer seasons and perhaps to inspire and console you through the winter. May they give you many years of enjoyment and help you towards your own deepening friendship with the plants that surround us and give us so much.

North Lincolnshire, 2019

Summer

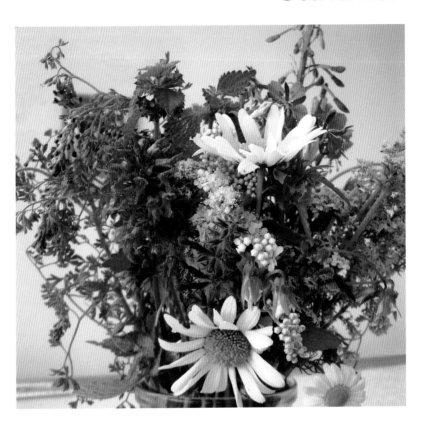

Introduction:
foraging and medicine making

Foraging

The subject of foraging can be a tricky and somewhat thorny one in this day and age, as so many people are rediscovering the joys of gathering their own food and medicines. This is, by necessity, a brief introduction to the topic, as well as a commentary on my own thoughts about it.

We live in a world that relies on increasing amounts of chemicals to get crops growing – so, unless you happen to live on or have access to organic farmland, I recommend that you don't gather from field margins, as there is no telling what the farmers may have sprayed on their crops. Many of our native medicines used to grow merrily in among the wheat and corn. Sadly, most of these are becoming increasingly rare in the wild, so I suggest that if you have a small bit of land, or even a yard and some pots, try growing some of them for yourselves. Cornflowers, chamomile and red poppies, in particular, make a merry display sown in tubs that can be freely moved around the yard or garden.

If you are gathering from the wild, try to pick from areas that are free from pollution, be it airborne or animal-borne – dog wee, for example, doesn't make good seasoning! Gather above dog height if at all possible, and if you are aiming to dry your herbs, gather them on a dry day, once the dew has evaporated. Pick only healthy plants, with no spots, fungus or withered bits – look for good, green foliage, and pick only a third of what is there. As a rule of thumb, if you can see where you have been, you have almost certainly gathered too much! I have seen elders, for example, stripped bare of flowers and fruit: this sort of behaviour is to be frowned upon, as is the arrogant assumption that the plants were put here for our benefit. They were not. We are all essentially equal, and it is a symbiotic relationship that we should all be working towards. Stripping the land of a particular plant is not neighbourly behaviour, after all! This is true even more in any heavily farmed counties or areas, where native wild flowers will be a rarer sight.

Drying and storing herbs

When you have gleefully lugged your harvest home, the next task is to bundle them up. To dry herbs, I recommend that you tie them in bunches of up to 12 stems, then hang them in a cool, well-ventilated room that doesn't get too much direct sunlight. This is especially true of aromatic plants, as those dried in hot temperatures will lose much of the volatile oils that make them smell and taste so good. Smaller bits of plants, leaves and flowers can be dried in baskets and are easy enough to turn over every day, either by hand or by giving the basket a gentle shake. Plants are dry when they break reasonably easily: they should still look like their fresh versions, just smaller and more desiccated. If, when you have finished, a plant looks grey or brown and doesn't smell of much or actively smells bad, it hasn't dried properly and should be composted.

These days I tend to recommend bunching herbs up using elastic bands – not as pretty as using garden twine, but, as plants dry, they shrink. It can be rather vexing coming downstairs in the morning and discovering that your carefully bunched herbs have all dropped out of their twine and are now happily mingled on the kitchen floor! While providing an excellent test for your budding skills in identifying plants by scent and look even while half-dried, it can be a frustrating enterprise trying to bunch them all up correctly again. Don't be afraid to experiment with finding the best room to dry your herbs in – if you have three possible rooms that might work, hang small bunches of herbs in each and monitor which gives you the best results. Remember that if it doesn't work the first time, you can always compost your plants and try again.

Seeds can be gathered from plants once they are going brown, or earlier if you prefer, while they are still green but fully formed. I tend to bunch them up with a paper bag tied over the heads and hang them upside down from the airer. The seeds will dry and gradually drop off, into the bag, after which they can be stored. Some can be used for the following year, others can be tinctured or used in teas or cooking. Remember to check whether the seed you want to work with is better used fresh. Also, if you want to grow some herbs from your own seed, check which of these will do better planted directly from the parent plant and which need to be stored before sowing. Angelica, for example, doesn't store well, so if you want to propagate your angelica plants, you will need to plant the seeds as soon as you gather them.

To store your herbs, clean, dry glass jars work well – a little time spent on labelling can make the resulting jars look beautiful. Chop the herbs using kitchen scissors, and pack them into jars, labelling them carefully with their English and Latin names and the date. Bear in mind that the smaller your herbs have been chopped, the larger the surface area exposed to air, which means they may not last quite as long. I tend to store my herbs in larger pieces and chop them later, according to need. It does make for more work, but the herbs store better and for longer. Dried herbs should be stored out of direct sunlight: mine are on a shelf in a shady kitchen that rarely gets direct sunlight, a situation that works well. Dried herbs will usually last up to two years, though it does vary fairly widely between herbs – I have had some that are perfectly good after three years, and others that lose their virtue in one. Go by eye, scent and taste – if it looks and smells good and still has a strong, vibrant flavour, it will almost certainly still be absolutely fine to use. If it has faded and doesn't taste or smell of much, compost it.

Root and bark, which are best dried in a dehydrator or low oven, are more commonly gathered in spring and in autumn, so more on this subject can be found in the other two books in the series.

Medicine making

Medicine making can be quite an art in and of itself. There is a plethora of superb books on the subject, some of which I have included in the bibliography. I do a lot of medicine making, and I feel that there is a huge overlap between medicine and food – so this book contains medicines, yes, but also wild-food recipes where appropriate. I encourage you to have a go at making your own medicines and wild foods – the enterprise can be time-consuming sometimes, but ultimately it is extremely rewarding. There is nothing like using your own hand-made creams to ease sunburn or bites and stings, or enjoying your own herbal teas from the garden! Better yet, you have full control over exactly what ingredients you use, so you can be sure that your hand-made products are all completely natural.

Equipment

There are a few pieces of equipment I strongly recommend you try to obtain if you plan to do much medicine making.

Kilner-type jars with a rubber seal are a must for tincture making, as is a mezzaluna – a semi-circular chopping knife; these little blades can make short work of a pile of herbs and are very satisfying to use. A double boiler is another must-have piece of kit for making infused oils and balms. Try, if possible, to have a set of wooden spoons and pans just for medicine making. Don't use aluminium pans, as aluminium tends to leech into the medicines: go, instead, for stainless steel, ceramic or toughened glass.

A measuring jug and a set of measuring spoons are also handy. Spoons that go up in increments of ¼–½ teaspoons are most useful, as these also make very good dosage cups. Keeping a metre or so of medium-weave cheesecloth in the cupboard is another trick I highly recommend – this will come in handy for all kinds of straining and can also be used for plaisters. If you have old tea towels that are towards the end of their useful life, save a few for plaisters and poultices.

Lastly, a rough-sided mortar and pestle is a must. Smooth-sided sets are great for certain jobs, but for really pulverising herbs and seeds a good, heavy, rough-sided set is invaluable. Most of this equipment can be found in second-hand shops if you keep an eye out, or in good kitchen hardware stores.

Teas and decoctions

Teas, or tisanes, are essentially an infusion, in hot water, of one or more herbs, either dried or fresh. Most herb teas and tisanes can be drunk up to three times a day, and they are very simple to make. If you are using fresh herbs, allow 1–2 heaped teaspoons of the fresh herb, chopped, to a cup of hot water. If you are using dried herbs, one gently heaped teaspoon is usually enough. Remember that fresh herbs have a much higher water content, which makes them more bulky. If you are brewing aromatic herbs, remember to cover the pot as the tea brews, otherwise the essential oils will evaporate; this is rather a shame, as it is these compounds that make the tea taste good and also provide a lot of the medicinal virtues.

Teas can be drunk as is, sweetened with honey and sliced fruit, or used as a skin wash or bath. They don't tend to keep well, so I recommend making and drinking your tea over the course of a day. You can make teas in cups or jugs, cafetieres or teapots, or you can make your own small muslin tea sacks to infuse the herbs in.

Cold infusions are effectively just cold water poured over chopped herbs in a Kilner jar, which is then stored in the fridge overnight while the herbs infuse. This suits very well herbs with a high mucilage content, as this is usually destroyed by heat and doesn't extract very well in alcohol. In my experience, this method is best for fresh herbs, such as marshmallow leaf or root. Nettle leaf also makes a lovely cold infusion.

Decoctions are a little more complicated, but not overly so: these consist basically of herbs that have been boiled in water until the water content has reduced by around one third of its total volume. The method lends itself well to fruit, bark, seeds and woody bits of the herbs, as the water will have more time to extract the properties of the herb and, as the water molecules are driven with much more force against the sides of the plant matter, it will do a better job of extracting useful properties. Decoctions can be either short: boiled for a fairly brief amount of time, but with the result that they will only keep for a shorter time in the fridge, or long: boiled for a number of hours with regular water top-ups, and therefore able to be kept for much a longer time if kept refrigerated.

Decoctions can be used in much the same way as teas, but with much lower dosages: about 50 ml (1¾ fl oz), two to three times a day, usually works well, though this is highly dependent on the herbs used.

Syrups and honeys

Syrups are the product of an infusion or decoction mixed with sugar as a preservative. These lend themselves well to fruit such as elderberries, or combinations such as thyme and liquorice as a cough syrup; they can be a much more palatable way to get herbs into children and more fussy adults. Syrups require a large quantity of sugar to really preserve them and can sometimes go mouldy. Unfortunately they do need actual sugar, as it acts as a preservative, so honey will not suffice. If you really don't want much or any sugar, I recommend making up a decoction or infusion sweetened as you choose, then freezing it in ice-cube trays. When you need the herbs, take out a cube, pop it into a glass of water, then drink.

Herbal honeys can be made by finely chopping fresh herbs and stirring them into a jar of honey. Local honey is best, if you can find it, as you can never be too sure what has gone into most of the honeys found on supermarket shelves. Herbal honeys have the advantage that a teaspoon contains the herb as well as the honey, giving them a wide variety of applications – topical for wounds, grazes and stings, or as part of the diet, stirred into herbal teas, used to make drinks at the weekend – the possibilities are extensive! They will usually keep for at least a year, provided the herbs are surface dry when you chop them, so that you have not introduced too much extra water into the blend.

Tinctures, elixirs and honegars

These are all made in similar ways and usually involve either alcohol or vinegar – I usually recommend unpasteurised cider vinegar. They have the advantage that they will often preserve the herbs for much longer periods, and only a small dose is needed to be medicinally effective. A teaspoon of a vile-tasting tincture may, after all, be a more palatable option than a whole cupful of an equally foul-tasting tea. It also has the advantage of speed for those with a busy lifestyle. I do recommend where possible trying to keep both tea and tincture in the cupboard – in this busy modern world we all live far too fast, and slowing down enough to take the time to make and drink a cup of healing tea is as much a part of the medicine as the herbs themselves.

Tinctures and elixirs are basically herbs chopped and infused in alcohol. In the case of an elixir, a form of sweetener has been added, usually honey, but I have also used maple syrup perfectly well. To make a cottage tincture, just chop plenty of the fresh or dried herb, pack it into a jar and pour over the alcohol, allowing an extra 1.25 cm (½ in.) of liquid on top of the herb. Let the whole lot steep for at least a fortnight, then strain and bottle, labelling carefully with the English and Latin names and the date of bottling. Be aware that the stronger the alcohol, the longer the tincture will last. Also, if you use fresh herbs, remember that the extra water content in the herbs will dilute the tincture. For a stronger tincture, wilt the herbs for a few days beforehand, or dry them entirely. If you are making an elixir, just add honey along with the herbs.

Honegars are made in much the same way, but using unpasteurised cider vinegar instead of alcohol, also with herbs and honey.

Throughout this book, I have included many recipes for tinctures, elixirs and honegars, each of which will, hopefully, clearly explain the process in detail for those of you who fancy having a go. Specific instructions are provided for individual plants. Some instructions may seem repeated from herb to herb – this is to remove the need to flip back and forth in the book.

Infused oils, creams and salves

Infused oils can be made with a huge range of leaves and flowers from the hedgerow or herb garden; there are two main ways of going about this.

Sun-infused oils are effectively just the flowers, picked on a dry day and packed into a glass jar, with organic seed oil poured over. A piece of cloth or kitchen roll is tied onto the top to allow water to evaporate and to stop beasties from getting in. The whole jar is then placed in the sun to infuse until the oil has changed colour. This can be rather exciting to watch, and a whole range of gorgeous coloured oils is possible, from calendula's vivid orange to St John's wort's rich red.

Hob-infused oils are usually made in a double boiler or a slow cooker, or in a bain marie in the oven. These, too, are simple to make: it involves placing the chopped herbs and the oil either into a double boiler or a slow cooker (I recommend having one especially for the purpose) or sealing them in a tin in a water bath in the oven. Over time, the oil gently heats and extracts the properties from the plant. Historically, infused oils were made by literally frying the herbs in the fat; however, having tried this with coconut oil and herbs, I'm not convinced this actually extracts and preserves the medicinal properties of the plant, as the higher level of heat tends to break down some of the more delicate plant constituents. Using the slower methods mentioned throughout this book certainly gives a surer result.

To avoid your oils going rancid, make sure the plants you use are completely dry to the touch, and if your oil looks rather murky once you've finished infusing it, just pop it into a clean, dry glass jar or jug and leave it for a day or two. The murky content will usually sink to the bottom of the jug, allowing you to pour off the clear oil. Do not bottle murky oil – it may go rancid and create a stench, which I recommend you avoid if at all possible!

Salves and ointments are made by adding beeswax in various proportions to the finished oil; creams are made by adding aromatic water as well as beeswax. I have included recipes for all three throughout the book, so I won't go into detail about them here.

Summer herbs for the medicine garden

Growing your own herbs is a pleasure and a delight that I highly recommend to anyone with just a small amount of space. You don't even really need a garden – a corner of a yard, a space outside your front door, a balcony or even window boxes will give you the scope to grow a plethora of fantastically useful plants.

Below are listed a few of the plants that I most recommend; they are mentioned in more detail in the book, along with a few notes on growing and caring for them, in the hope that it will encourage you to have a go at growing your own. I've grown all of these plants in a variety of different circumstances, from pots to tiny yards to full-sized gardens, and I can attest to their versatility and ease to grow.

First on the list would have to be **agrimony** (*Agrimonia eupatoria*), simply because it has such a wide range of useful properties, as well as being an exceptionally pretty wild plant in its own right. I've easily grown agrimony in pots, though it does do better in poor soil with a little benign neglect.

Next would have to be **calendula** (*Calendula officinalis*), which pretty much anyone can grow and which makes gloriously sunny displays of orange and yellow flowers all through the summer. The odd-shaped seeds can be sown from March through to June; once they have put on a bit of growth, they will reward you with a plethora of flowers for medicine for months on end. If you have a mild winter, you may find that you have flowers right the way through to December; they absolutely thrive in pots and are happy in most kinds of soil.

Elder (*Sambucus nigra*) is another noteworthy plant – often decried as a weed, this wonderfully useful shrub really deserves a place in every garden, even if it is the only tree you grow. Ignore the neighbours carping about it – with flowers, fruits, leaves and bark that can all be gathered for medicine, this is a shrub worth far more love than we give it. It will grow happily in large pots, as well as in the ground.

Next on the list: **honeysuckle** (*Lonicera periclymenum*). A beautiful, fragrant plant, which really does double duty as a stunning addition to the garden as well as providing medicine, this climbing plant can be scrambled up the sides of buildings, where it will provide a scented glory of flowers throughout the summer. Equally happy in shade as well as sun, honeysuckle is rampant in one of our local woods, where branches can often be found with the characteristic spiral groove running up it where honeysuckle has clung on. I used to have honey-suckle growing outside my bedroom window every summer, where in the evenings it would make each breath a perfumed delight.

Lady's mantle (*Alchemilla mollis / vulgaris*) produces tidy hummocks of leaves dewed with silver each morning, giving rise later on to lacy displays of pale-green flowers; with its medicinal purposes as well, it makes for a wonderful addition to the medicine garden. As easy to grow in pots as it is in the ground, this can be moved around the yard or will look beautiful flanking the front door in window boxes.

Meadowsweet (*Filipendula ulmaria*), with its stomach-settling properties, produces beautifully shaped leaves and, later in the season, plumes of creamy, highly scented flowers, which can be used in cooking as well as providing great medicine. This lovely plant likes to keep its feet wet if possible, so don't forget to water it regularly, especially if it is in a pot.

Self heal (*Prunella vulgaris*), a low-growing perennial, provides unobtrusive ground cover and, later in the summer, purple flowers much beloved by bees. Why not grow it underneath your elder tree? It can also be tucked into window boxes to provide an intriguing foil to larger plants, or around the base of larger plants growing in tubs.

St John's wort (*Hypericum perforatum*) will readily self-seed everywhere if given half a chance, and what better reason to make sure you make full use of those sunny yellow flowers in the summer? Thriving happily in pots or in the ground, this beautiful plant provides a striking feature set against walls, especially in late summer, when the leaves begin to take on red tones.

This is the barest introduction to herbs for a fledgling wild medicine garden – there are more in the other books in the series: *Wild Medicine: Autumn and Winter* and *Wild Medicine: Spring*.

Now, without further ado, let me introduce a few of the herbs, those fascinating denizens of hedgerow and garden, myth and dream. Bear in mind that most of them can be obtained from specialist garden centres or herb nurseries and will often grow very happily in a garden, so if you are concerned about gathering from the wild, this need not deter you from growing your own and gathering from an environment you know and are certain about.

Agrimony
Agrimonia eupatoria

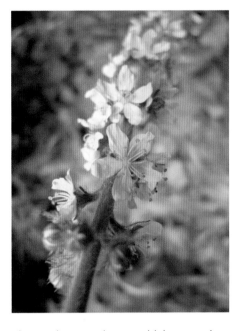

Also known as: church steeples, tea plant, cocklebur, garclive, philanthropos, little cocklebur, fur-burr, catch-as-catch-can, liverwort, sticklewort, stickwort, umakhuthula, ntola

Family Rosaceae.

Habitat and description Agrimony is a low-growing perennial with a long history of use in the UK and Europe. The leaves are rich green on top and silvery-coloured underneath, a little over 10 cm (4 in.) in length, with five or more opposing pairs of toothed leaflets. The small yellow flowers with five yellow petals appear on tall stems. The stems themselves are slightly hairy, much like the leaves, and have small, round,

15

ribbed fruits with hooked bristles that stick to things really easily – hence a lot of the folk names for the plant. If you have pets, expect them to bring the seeds in on their fur, and if you go out in a long skirt, expect to come back adorned with seed heads! The seed pods contain two seeds each.

The plant likes to grow in well-drained soil. The flowers always smell of apricot, and I have noticed that even the leaves have a scent of it when grown in plenty of sun. The plant can be propagated by root division in the autumn and also grows readily from seed. I have recently found agrimony growing on roadside verges and around the bases of old trees where the grass doesn't come through as thickly and where it is often deposited by birds and creatures who carry away the prickly seeds in the autumn. It can also be seen in field edges, open grassland, railway margins and waste ground. It can be found in meadows and woodland edges as well as happily tucking itself in around tree bases.

Where to find it   Most temperate regions, including the UK and Ireland; Europe, even places like Russia and some of the Scandinavian countries; North America; parts of Africa and Asia.

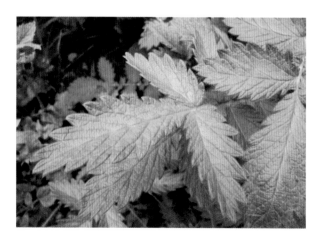

Parts used   The whole herb, which is gathered when the plant is in flower.

When to gather   July and August.

Medicines to make   Agrimony tea, tincture and elixir for liver and kidney health; agrimony salve or cream for bruises, bumps and cuts; agrimony cider vinegar for sunburn.

Constituents   Lots of lovely tannins, both condensed and hydrolysable, 3%–21%, depending on the plant and where it has grown; flavonoids, including glucosides of luteolin, quercetin and apigenin; volatile oils; some triterpenes, coumarin, glycosidal bitters and salicylic acid.

Planetary influence   Jupiter.

Associated deities and heroes   None known at present – perhaps do some testing and decide for yourself which deity or deities this herb could be associated with.

Constitution   Cool and dry.

Actions and indications   Agrimony is a particularly good herb for issues related to the digestive system as well as to the urinary tract, being well suited to the treatment of inflamed, weepy conditions of the body.

In the digestive system, agrimony is handy for treating constipation and diarrhoea, especially where these conditions alternate, indicating lax, irritated tissues. It is also good for the liver and related organs, coordinating the function of the whole digestive tract. It is useful for the relief of jaundice and can be used to clear congestion in the liver, with its related symptoms of appetite loss, poor digestion and pain in the right side. It can be used, alongside a low-fat diet, to treat fatty liver brought on by overindulgence; it combines well with dandelion root and milk thistle if treating this disorder.

It is not recommended that it be used to treat constipation where this is not present with alternating diarrhoea, because it is astringent and could worsen the problem, though it could be useful for treating constipation due to an over-relaxed bowel tract: examining the pattern and nature of the constipation would be necessary in determining this. Agrimony is regarded as being a specific for children's diarrhoea and has been used to relieve early-stage appendicitis. An infusion of agrimony can be used to ease gastritis and as part of a treatment for Irritable Bowel Syndrome (IBS).

For the urinary tract, agrimony is good for kidney-stone-related pain, cystitis and irritable bladder; it can be used for children who are bedwetting and getting worried about potty training, as well as for adults struggling with incontinence – again, this is due in part to the tannin content.

Agrimony is also an excellent topical skin herb, with the tincture being very good for burns. The whole herb is handy for stopping bleeding and easing pain. It makes a very useful ointment for wounds and bruises and can also be used as a gargle to relieve sore throats (probably even better with a little honey added for this purpose!).

As a mild remedy for the lungs, it can be used to treat bronchitis and any lung illness that causes excessive production of phlegm, as well as to ease asthma. Because the plant is an astringent, it can be used to dry up excessive fluids of most kinds, including excessive menstrual bleeding, and to ease and stop bleeding from injuries.

It can be used to ease feverish conditions and reduce inflammation, making it useful for inflammation of the urinary tract and problems relating to the liver and gall bladder, and it is a useful addition to medicines for general inflammatory conditions.

Agrimony is a valuable addition to the herb garden as well as to the home herbalist's pharmacy, because, alongside a gentle nature, it has such a wide variety of applications.

Folklore   It was believed that the herb could treat all eye disorders – a belief that led to the name 'agrimony', derived from 'agremone', meaning 'white speck on the eye'. The second half of the name comes from the King of Pontus, Mithridates Eupator, who was, according to legend, the first to discover how this plant could be used in medicine. There is, however, some doubt as to whether he was referring to agrimony at all: he may actually have been talking about a totally different species – *Eupatorium cannabinum*, or hemp agrimony. Either way, agrimony does have an impressive history of use, dating back to Dioscorides.

Agrimony has a long-standing reputation as a useful plant to heal snake bite and to ward off malevolent elves and pixies. The Anglo-Saxons added it to their Holy Salve to avert all kinds of unpleasantness. Medieval monks used to grow agrimony in their gardens to treat wounds and stomach problems. It was also used by the Native Americans as a fever remedy, and the French used it in their *eau de arquebusade*, created to treat battle wounds in the fifteenth century.

Dose   Up to 4 ml (¾ tsp) of the tincture three times a day, or 1 cup of boiling water infused with up to 2 tsp of the dried herb, drunk three times a day.

Contraindications   No contraindications found thus far, though given that the plant contains coumarins, I would recommend some caution if you are taking anticoagulant drugs such as warfarin – better safe than sorry!

Agrimony recipes

Agrimony tea

This tea is very easy to make, ideally with fresh leaves from the garden, but the dried herb also works perfectly well. If using fresh herbs, allow 1–2 heaped teaspoons of the chopped herb per mug of boiling water. For dried herbs, one slightly heaped teaspoon should be plenty. Pour over water that is just off the boil and allow it to steep for 5–10 minutes, then drink. This can be sweetened with honey as desired, or flavoured with a slice of lemon if preferred. Drink up to three times a day as a tonic for over-relaxed, inflamed mucous membranes wherever they are sited in the body, or as a tonic for the kidneys.

Agrimony-infused oil and salve

Ingredients

- » minimum ½ pint of loosely packed leaves and flowering stems, or just leaves if picked before flowering (if using dried herbs, choose organic if possible, and always use herbs with a good, green colour to them)
- » organic seed oil: rapeseed, sunflower, sweet almond all work well

For the salve:

- » beeswax pellets: 12 g per 100 ml (3½ fl oz) of oil
- » essential oils, as preferred – lavender, frankincense or chamomile all work beautifully (if you are using lavender, you can even add the flowers to the original infused oil instead of including essential oil drops)

Instructions   Gather the herbs on a dry day, once the sun has been on them for long enough to dry off any dew or rain: if damp gets into the oil, it could make it rancid. Using a mezza-luna, sharp scissors or a knife, chop the herbs finely, having first checked them for insects or bird poop. Pack them into the top of a double boiler and pour over enough of the oil to just cover the herbs, either fresh or dried, so that you can see a thin skin of oil on top of the leaf matter. Fill the saucepan at the base with water and put the whole thing on a moderate simmer, leaving it to steep for at least half an hour. If you want a particularly strong oil, strain out the first lot of herbs, and add a second lot. You can steep the herbs for as long as you would like – but make sure the base of the pan doesn't boil dry and keep an eye on the colour of the oil itself. Once the oil is as strong as desired, strain out the herbs through muslin or a piece of kitchen roll, and pour the oil into a clean, dry Pyrex or glass jug. Let it settle for a while if there is any concern about water content, then pour off the clear oil into a clean, dry glass bottle.

To make the salve: To each 100 ml (3½ fl oz) of the infused oil, add 12 g of beeswax pellets, putting both ingredients into the top pan of a double boiler. Bring to a gentle simmer, stirring until the beeswax pellets have dissolved, then turn off the heat and add the essential oil drops: 5 drops per 100 ml usually works well. Stir again briefly, then pour the resulting salve into clean glass jars; once cool, label the jars with the name of the salve and when it was made. This salve can be used on minor scrapes, cuts and bumps. It will store for at least a year if kept out of direct sunlight.

Agrimony cottage tincture or elixir

Ingredients / equipment
- » plenty of fresh or dried agrimony leaves
- » brandy or vodka, or unpasteurised cider vinegar
- » local honey, if preferred
- » one 1-litre resealable jar

Instructions   As with the previous recipe, make sure the plant matter is clean and free from bugs and pests, then chop it thoroughly, looking to get pieces no larger and preferably smaller than your little fingernail. Pack it into the jar and pour over enough alcohol or vinegar to cover the herbs plus an extra 2.5–4 cm (1–1½ in.) on top, then stir in at least 12 ml (one dessertspoonful) of honey – liquid honey works well for this recipe and is easier to work with than set honey. Put the lid on the jar and shake it up thoroughly; press the herbs back down with a spoon, then let the whole thing settle for several weeks, shaking it up every couple of days and repeating the packing down of the plant matter. Finally, strain out the herbs, and take 10 ml (2 tsp) up to three times a day as a gentle tonic for the digestion and kidneys.

Black horehound
Ballota nigra / Marrubium nigrum

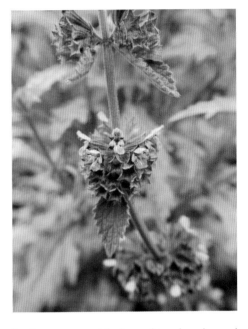

Also known as: black stinking horehound

Family Lamiaceae.

Habitat and description This really rather unpleasant-smelling perennial can often be found growing by the wayside, near hedgerows and on wasteland, where it can bush out into surprising clumps of plant growth. It is quite easily cultivated in the herb garden as well, though it tends to be a bit of a thug – seemingly a characteristic of many of the herbs in the lamiaceae family, all of which have a strong survival instinct. Once the plant is well grown, it is rather attractive, particularly when it is in flower and surrounded by bees.

The plant grows up to 30 cm (1 ft) tall and has slightly murky-green, roughly spear-shaped, toothed leaves arranged in pairs on the typical square stem, much of which is lightly furred. The flowers form in whorls and are deep pinky purple, with the characteristic lip. Black horehound is part of the same plant family as deadnettle, mint, skullcap and assorted others and possesses many of the same family characteristics of square stem and similar leaf shape and flower structure. Black horehound likes to grow on waste ground and will often be found growing on freshly turned earth. I have found that it doesn't like too easy a time of it – planted in fertile soil, it will often die off.

Where to find it   Native to Asia and the Mediterranean, like so many of the plants high in volatile oils, it has naturalised

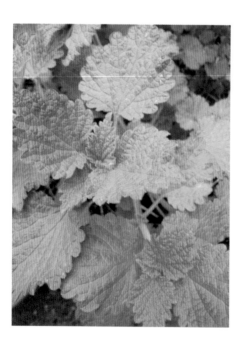

around most of the world, seeming to prefer temperate to warm areas. It can be found in New Zealand and Eastern USA, as well as throughout most of Europe.

Parts used   Aerial parts.

When to gather   June through to September, when in flower.

Medicines to make   Tinctures, pills and elixirs for nausea; dry, as a tea for diarrhoea; infused into oil.

Constituents   The plant contains diterpenoids, such as marrubiin and ballonigrin, and antibacterial phenylpropanoids, plus, of course, volatile oils and flavonoids.

Planetary influence   Mercury.

Associated deities   None known at present.

Constitution   Warm and dry.

Actions and indications   One of black horehound's primary and most useful actions is as an anti-emetic, especially for morning sickness during pregnancy and for travel or motion sickness – it combines well with ginger, raspberry leaf and / or chamomile for both purposes. It can also be used to treat persistent and ongoing diarrhoea, especially where this is combined with trembling, weakness and general debility, though these last two would not be surprising, really – I rather suspect anyone who had suffered from diarrhoea for more than a couple of days would feel as if they had been put through a wringer, regardless of any other symptoms! The diarrhoea this is well suited to emerges without warning and is not necessarily due to food not well tolerated or that has, perhaps, gone off.

Black horehound can also be used to treat a range of digestive complaints, such as dyspepsia and flatulence; it is particularly good for treating digestive upset and vomiting where this is of nervous origin. It is perhaps on a par with vervain for this, though I have found that vervain often suits people of a warm constitution and black horehound those of a colder constitution. Add it to recipes or prescriptions for those whose nerves cause significant digestive upset.

It also has some actions on the respiratory tract as an antispasmodic, making it useful in the treatment of bronchitis and asthma, as well as of chronic coughs – it can be combined with demulcents such as marshmallow leaf or plantain leaf for this purpose and will work alongside these two to encourage mucus to thin to normal levels, while paring back the production levels.

It can also be used as an emmenagogue to bring on periods delayed due to nervous tension, as well as to dry up excessive menstrual bleeding and normalise the menstrual cycle. By extension, it can also be combined with other herbs to ease labour pains.

Folklore   The Latin name *Ballota* derives from *ballo*, meaning 'to reject', indicating that cattle will not eat it (not surprising, either, given how unpleasant it smells)! Very little other folklore seems to exist for this plant, which seems odd, considering that it was known by Dioscorides and other notables of Greek medicine.

Dose   Up to 4 g of the dried herb three times a day or related tincture dose – approximately 2 ml (½ tsp) three times a day. As is the case with most herbs, dosage really depends on what you are trying to accomplish – smaller doses are more tonic, larger doses are more heroic.

Contraindications   Do not use during pregnancy unless under the guidance of a medical herbalist.

Black horehound recipes

Ginger, chamomile and black horehound elixir for nausea and vomiting

Ingredients

» 2½ cm (1 in.) piece of fresh root ginger or ½ tsp dried ginger
» 2 tbsp fresh, or 1 tbsp dried German chamomile
» 2 tbsp fresh, or 1 tbsp dried black horehound
» brandy
» honey

Instructions Finely dice the fresh root ginger and the fresh herbs; if you are using dried herbs, make sure they are chopped up finely enough, using kitchen scissors if need be. Pile the ingredients into a Kilner jar and pour over enough brandy to cover the herbs, with an extra 2.5 cm (1 in.) on top, then stir in 2 large tbsp of local honey. Put the lid on and shake up the jar, then leave it to steep for a fortnight. Take 5 ml (1 tsp) in a little water to relieve nausea and vomiting. This mix is suitable for travel sickness and, in small doses, also for morning sickness. It will also work beautifully for those struggling with nausea of a nervous cause – exam nerves, for example. You can multiply up the quantities of herbs used to make larger batches.

Black horehound and peppermint pills

Ingredients

» fresh or dried peppermint leaves
» fresh or dried black horehound leaves
» local runny honey
» arrowroot powder

Instructions   Finely chop the fresh herbs into the smallest pieces you can manage – a mezzaluna is really useful here, or, if you are making a large batch, a nutribullet might help, though you may lose some of the juice that way! You can also use dried herbs for this recipe – if you go down this route, powder them as much as you possibly can in a rough-sided mortar and pestle first. Pour the finely chopped herbs into a bowl and add a large tablespoonful of the runny honey, using the back of a spoon to work the herbs carefully into the honey. Add one large tablespoonful of arrowroot and mix this into the sticky concoction thoroughly, until you get a consistency that can be rolled into little balls; keep adding more arrowroot until the desired consistency is reached. Roll the pills into small balls about the size of a pea, coat them in arrowroot, put them on a layer of greaseproof paper and place them either in the oven on a low temperature or in a dehydrator. Once these have dried out, they can be stored in an airtight jar; stored out of sunlight, they will last some time. Take up to three pills for nausea or upset stomach, chewing them up before swallowing.

Black horehound and plantain cough syrup

Ingredients
- » 10 stems of fresh black horehound
- » 20 large leaves of ribwort plantain
- » 2 large organic lemons
- » 2½-cm (1-in.) piece of fresh ginger root
- » 1 whole star anise
- » 500 ml (17½ fl oz) water
- » 500 g (1 lb 1½ oz) sugar

Instructions   Thoroughly chop the two herbs and pile them into a saucepan, along with the zest and juice of the lemons, the pulverised star anise and the grated ginger root. Pour over the water and bring to a gentle simmer, keeping the pot covered. Simmer for at least 10 minutes, cool slightly, and filter the syrup blend through a muslin cloth; then put the liquid back into the clean pan, along with the sugar. Bring to a gentle simmer again, stirring regularly until the sugar has dissolved, then bring to a boil; boil for 5 minutes, keeping a close eye on it to make sure it doesn't burn. Use a funnel to pour the hot syrup into clean glass storage bottles – preferably ones designed to cope with hot beverages, as some bottles will break when you introduce hot liquids into them. Put the tops on and turn the bottles upside down briefly, to sterilise the necks of the bottles again and to encourage the lids to form a good seal. This syrup will keep for up to three months in the fridge and can be taken in doses of 15 ml (1 tbsp) up to three times a day to soothe coughs and encourage expectoration and removal of phlegm.

Calendula
Calendula officinalis

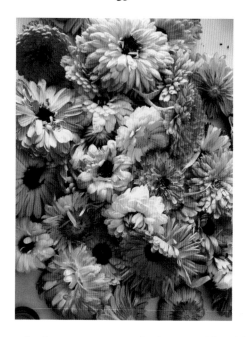

Also known as: marybud, marigold, gold-bloom, summer's bride, husbandman's dial, holigold, bride of the sun, spousa solis, gold, golds, the sun's gold, ball's eyes, bees-love, oculis christi, drunkard, marygold, mary gowles, ruddles, ruddes, solis sponsa, solsequia

Family Asteraceae.

Habitat and description While not strictly a wild flower, I have seen this self-sown and naturalised often enough to include it here. Calendula is an annual, commonly grown in the garden from seed, with resiny, mid- to light-green oval-shaped leaves and large, many-petalled flower heads that range from rich orange to yellow gold, depending on the type of calendula cultivated. It likes plenty of sun, appropriately enough, and prefers a reasonably well-drained soil. Calendula has been a popular garden flower for many years and has a well-deserved reputation – it is beautiful and useful in equal measure and will self-sow very readily around the garden. The seeds are quite distinctive: curved, pale brown and rough-textured; they keep very well from one year to the next if kept dry.

It is named calendula for its tendency to flower pretty much every month of the year, given the right conditions, and will thrive just as much in pots as it does in the garden, creating a sunny golden orange array much beloved by bees and butterflies.

Where to find it   Originally from the Mediterranean region, calendula can be grown in most temperate to warm regions of the world, ranging from the UK and Europe to Asia and parts of the USA, Mexico and the Middle East, to name but a few.

Parts used   The flowers and leaves.

When to gather   June through September, on hot, sunny afternoons.

Medicines to make   Infused oils and salves, ointments, compresses, baths and washes for skin problems, cuts, grazes, bites and stings; tinctures and elixirs for skin and liver issues.

Constituents   Triterpenes; pentacyclic alcohols; flavonoids, including rutin; resins; saponins; sesquiterpene glycosides; volatile oils and polysaccharides; bitters, phytosterols, mucilage, carotenoids such as carotene and calendulin.

Planetary influence   The sun.

Associated deities and heroes   Sun Gods, and probably Goddesses as well – so Zeus, Apollo and other similar deities from various different cultures, as well as Amaterasu and suchlike; it is also sacred to the Aztec Goddess Xochiquetzal.

Festival Midsummer, Samhain.

Constitution Warm and dry.

Actions and indications Calendula is perhaps one of the most versatile and well-known herbs in the herbalist's arsenal. Externally it makes a fantastic wound and skin-condition herb, stopping bleeding and acting as an antiseptic when applied as a tincture or cream to wounds. It is particularly good on infected wounds, cleansing the injury and slowly removing the pus – in this sort of scenario I would recommend the patient to take it internally in addition to applying it to the wound, to help the lymph system deal with any potential infection. When used externally in this way, it also lessens scar formation and can benefit the appearance of keloid scars.

It is also useful on insect bites and sunburn as well as on scratches that are likely to be dirty, such as those caused

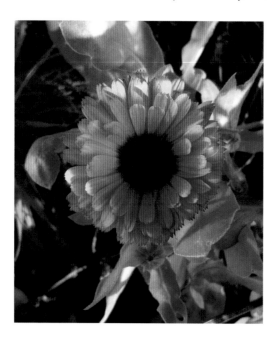

by cats or by brambles and other thorny shrubs and plants. Lastly, calendula is good for rashes, especially those caused by warm, damp weather, and can be useful in the treatment of thrush. Basically, for anything wrong with the skin – wounds, cuts, sores, rashes and suchlike – calendula is your herb. Two forms of the tincture are generally available – calendula in 90% alcohol, and calendula in 25% alcohol. The 90% tincture is usually used topically, and the 25% internally. To treat bleeding gums and gum disease, use a diluted tincture-and-water mix (50/50 works well); rinse the mouth with this twice a day, or soak a cotton wool pad in the mixture, squeeze out the excess, and tuck the pad between the affected gums and the side of the mouth for 30 minutes a day. If you are feeling brave, the same mixture can be used to treat stubborn instances of oral or vaginal thrush.

Internally, the plant works well with the lymph glands and can resolve lingering infections, soothe swollen glands and cleanse the lymph system as a whole, making it a valuable herb for those suffering from eruptive skin conditions such as acne, psoriasis and eczema – this is particularly true in the case of those with impaired liver function that is causing or worsening the skin disorder.

It also acts on the digestive system and is particularly useful in the treatment of illnesses caused by damaged or impaired liver function, as it lowers high enzyme counts caused by this. This makes it useful in the treatment of jaundice, hepatitis and cirrhosis, as well as being soothing to mucous membranes around the whole body, including the digestive system. It is warming and settling to the stomach and can be used to treat gastric ulceration, though I would recommend caution in this case, as I have noticed that ulceration of the digestive system often seems to be an overheated condition that may be exacerbated by using too much calendula. Consider combining it with one of the many useful demulcents for this – plantain or marshmallow works beautifully. Calendula can also be used to relieve jaundice and gall-bladder inflammation.

Calendula also acts as an emmenagogue, promoting the menses, as well as easing excessive period pain and normalising the cycle. The plant can be used to heal perineal tears from labour and cervical damage caused by abortion or miscarriage. It is extremely useful for those who struggle with premenstrual syndrome (PMS), as it eases the symptoms that cause irritability, bloating, water retention and skin problems (again, most likely due to its effect on the liver). It also makes a worthy ally in the treatment of pelvic congestion and any illnesses caused by this. During labour, calendula can be used to gently promote contractions and encourage delivery of the placenta.

It is also used as an all-round immune tonic and can ease fevers and measles, as well as making a fantastic eye bath for conjunctivitis – if you use it for this purpose, make sure you strain the tea through a coffee filter paper to remove any trace of dust or plant fragments.

Folklore   Old lore tells of the plant's use to grant a vision of anyone who has stolen anything from the bearer, as well as to engender a good reputation for the person.

An old love spell dictates that a woman should collect soil that her prospective partner has stepped on and pot it up with a calendula plant. The health of the plant indicates the health of the relationship. (The fact that the plant is an annual makes this somewhat suspect, if you ask me!)

The name of the plant derives from the Latin word *calends* or *kalendae*, the root word of 'calender' and originally a term for the first day of every month. Throughout the ancient world, in Egypt, Persia and Greece, as well as India, the plant had a wide range of uses ranging from medicine, to cookery, to devotional uses as altar decorations.

In Mexican lore, the plants grew where the blood of the native Mexicans had fallen when they were slaughtered by the invading Spanish conquistadors. The plant was sacred to the Goddess Xochiquetzal, Goddess of love, marriage and prostitutes as well as the patron of spinning, weaving, music, painting and carving, magic, art and dance. She was also the Goddess of the land of the dead, which is perhaps one of the reasons why calendulas are offered on the Day of the Dead.

Dose   A tea made with 2 tsp of dried herb to a cup of hot water three times a day, or more often if you are using it as a bath or a wash. Of the tincture, up to 10 ml (2 tsp) a day, depending on what you are trying to treat. If used as part of a prescription, I would use no more than about 30 ml (2 tbsp) per week in a formula. You can use tiny doses of the really strong 90%-proof calendula internally, but we are talking literally 1 ml a day here when combined with other herbs. It is really strong and is best reserved for significant fungal issues, like candida overgrowth.

Contraindications   None known at present, but it bears mentioning that the plant is a member of the daisy family and, as such, could possibly cause skin irritation to anyone with an allergy to members of the daisy family. Opinion over its safety during pregnancy seems to be divided; however, given that it can be used to promote contractions during labour, I would recommend that you give it a miss and go for something else instead.

Calendula recipes

Calendula infused oil

Ingredients / equipment
- » plenty of fresh flowers, picked on a dry day
- » organic seed oil

» one large jar
» muslin or kitchen roll
» rubber band

Instructions   Check the flowers over fairly carefully – in the summer, many little black bugs tend to hide in all the nooks and crannies of calendula flowers, and it can be a good idea to try to get rid of them first. Try putting the flowers in a basket in a shady or dark room with one open, sunny window – often the bugs will very happily leave the flowers and migrate back outside into the sunshine. Leave the flowers for about an hour for the best likelihood of evicting unwanted bug life. Once you are pretty sure all the passengers have gone, pack the flowers into the jar loosely, not pressing them down too much – the oil needs to have plenty of space to slip between the flowers. Pour over enough oil to cover all of the flowers, using a knitting needle or the end of a spoon to move the flowers around a little and make sure the oil gets into all the little spaces. Press the flowers under the level of the oil and put the kitchen roll or muslin over the top, fastening it in place with the rubber band, then stand the jar in a warm place with plenty of sunlight. Sunny windowsills work beautifully, as does the greenhouse; on a really hot day, stand it on the patio or bench in full sun. The oil can vary quite a bit where infusing is concerned – sometimes it will only take an afternoon, or, on cooler days, it may take several days. Once finished, it will take on a rich amber colour, after which you can pour it through the kitchen roll or muslin into a large jug or bowl. If there is any murky stuff in the bottom of the jar, try to avoid pouring that part through, and let the clear oil sit for a day or two before you bottle it. Generally, water will sink to the bottom, allowing you to pour off the clear oil.

Calendula hand balm for gardeners and other hard-working hands

Ingredients
- » 100 ml (3½ fl oz) of calendula-infused oil
- » 10 g beeswax
- » lavender essential oil

Instructions   Measure the oil into the top of a double boiler and add the beeswax, letting the whole lot warm through gently until the beeswax has melted, then give it a good stir and add the lavender essential oil. I usually find that 10 drops is plenty – enough to give it a good healing effect without making it overpoweringly strongly scented. Stir the balm again briefly, and pour it into clean, dry glass jars. Don't be tempted to put in more than 12 g of beeswax per 100 ml of oil: the first recipe I tried, many years ago, was a calendula balm, and, with too much beeswax in it, it unfortunately set solid!

Calendula and plantain tincture for digestive tone

Ingredients
- » plenty of fresh calendula flowers
- » a roughly equal amount of fresh plantain leaves
- » ½ tsp cinnamon
- » brandy
- » local honey

Instructions   Wash and thoroughly chop the herbs and pile them into a large jar, sprinkling the cinnamon in as well, then pour over plenty of the brandy until the herbs are just covered. Stir in a good-sized dollop of honey, put the lid on, and shake it up thoroughly to make sure the honey and brandy emulsifies properly. Press the herbs back down again, and put the jar into a cool, dark cupboard to infuse for a few weeks. Once you are happy the herbs have infused enough, strain them out and pour the resulting infused brandy into a bottle. Take 5 ml (1 tsp) of the mixture three times a day to relieve long-standing digestive issues such as wind or bloating.

Cornflower
Centaurea cyanus

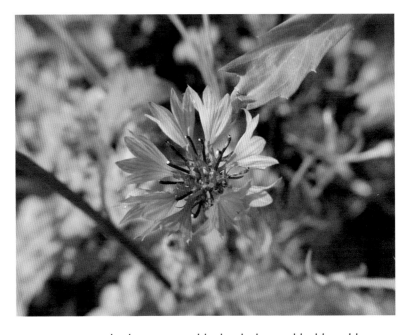

Also known as: bluebottle, hurtsickle, bluet, blue cap, bluebrow, cyanus

Family   Asteraceae.

Habitat and description   These charming blue flowers were commonly found growing at the edges of wheat- and corn-fields – hence the common name – up until we got into the habit of spraying herbicides on everything. Now, here in my native county of Lincolnshire, they can sometimes be found in field verges where farmers have planted them deliberately, and their reappearance is a welcome sight indeed! Corn-flowers are an annual, with globular-shaped flower heads featuring fairly distinctive blue petals that are summer-sky-coloured. The outer petals are tubular and trumpet-shaped, with lobes. They can sometimes be bought in wild-flower plant selections or are easy to grow from seed, thriving happily in most kinds of garden soil – indeed, there are a variety of cultivars that are grown for their decorative flower heads.

Cornflower usually starts as a fairly small, innocuous basal rosette of leaves but rapidly grows to form a sprawling, bushy annual with slender, straggly stems, lightly toothed upper leaves growing directly from the flower stems, and lower leaves that are more heavily lobed, much like the plant's knapweed relatives. The stem and leaves are covered in a light down coating. The flowers are prolific throughout the summer, and I have often found that the more you pick for medicine making, the more the plant will produce.

Where to find   Cornflower is native to Europe and the UK but has naturalised in many temperate regions of the world, including parts of Australia and the USA.

Parts used   Flowers; leaves have been used in the past to make decoctions.

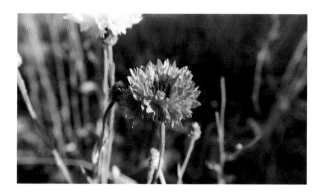

When to gather   All summer through – they flower from the end of May in warmer climes, right through to the end of September in mild years.

Medicines to make   Teas and tinctures for sleep and digestive purposes, skin washes, elixirs and salves; decoctions.

Constituents   Flavonoids, anthocyanin glycosides, sesquiterpene lactones and coumarins; also some polysaccharides, including glucose and galactose, and polyacetylenes.

Planetary influence   Saturn.

Associated deities and heroes   Flora, and most harvest Goddesses – for example, Demeter.

Festival   Lammas / Lughnasadh / Harvest.

Constitution   Cool and dry.

Actions and indications   The cornflower is a herb that has a long and venerable history of use but has rather fallen out of favour these days, perhaps owing to its rapid decline at the edge of cornfields. Culpeper used a powder of the leaves for bruises and contusions and had a very high opinion of the whole plant as being proof against many kinds of poisons, bites and plagues. The juice could be used to heal open wounds.

These days the flowers are used more often than the whole herb. They have a range of properties: taken internally, they are a tonic and stimulant to the whole digestive tract, including the liver and gall bladder, making them well suited to those with a very hot, over-active digestive system. The herb is a gentle laxative as well as being astringent, very useful for constipation due to an over-relaxed bowel system when accompanied by symptoms of heat, such as a red tongue or flushed face. The flowers are anti-inflammatory and cooling, with some febrifuge (fever-lowering) properties when drunk hot as a tea, and the decoction of the leaves has been used to relieve rheumatic conditions, perhaps due to their anti-inflammatory, tonic properties.

Cornflowers also have an affinity with the kidneys, acting as a gentle diuretic and tonic and regulating kidney performance. The plant has historically been linked with an increased resistance to infection and has been credited, as mentioned above, with being suited to many kinds of bites, stings and poisons, making it a great addition to healing balms and salves and, perhaps, in tonic blends to boost and improve immune response – consider combining it with elderberry, self heal and herb robert for this purpose.

I have most often used this herb as a gently calming, settling herb, very useful for anxiety attacks and over-stimulated nervous systems. It can help down-regulate the nervous system and ease up the fight-or-flight response, as well as to soothe hyper-alertness. It makes a pleasant tea to encourage a restful night's sleep, if drunk a couple of hours before bed. It also has a reputation as being useful for partial paralysis following strokes, perhaps owing in part to its tonic action on so many organs, gently encouraging the body towards better health and mopping up the damage done by the stroke along the way.

The whole herb is gently astringent and can be used externally for a variety of issues, including as a rinse, wash or cool compress for an inflamed scalp. A cool skin bath of it can be used for sunburn, bites and stings, and a salve can be used for cuts, grazes and stings. A compress of the decoction or the chopped plant matter can be used for infected wounds, to clean them out and encourage healing, as it is anti-fungal, antispasmodic and antibiotic; a tea of the flowers can be used for inflammation of the eye and for eye fatigue in general.

Folklore   Known as 'hurtsickle' because the tough stems used to blunt the hand sickles used for harvesting. Named Cyanus after a follower of the Flower Goddess Flora, and linked to the famous healer centaur Chiron. The French used to make a famous water for weak eyes using the flowers, which have long been linked to the eyes and to eyesight in general.

A juice of the petals can be used to make blue ink when mixed with alum, and it has been used historically in watercolour painting. Sadly it seems that the dye made with it is not colour-fast and cannot be used to dye clothes permanently.

The dried petals can be used in pot pourri to give colour – but make sure you dry them in the dark if using them for this purpose as they fade rapidly to a soft pinkish grey if dried in normal light levels.

Dose   A tea can be drunk up to three times a day, allowing 1 tsp of dried herb to a cup of hot water and infusing it for 5 minutes. Of the cottage tincture, 5 ml (1 tsp) three times a day should work well.

Contraindications   None found at present, but given it does have some nebulous links with the menstrual cycle, I would recommend avoiding it during pregnancy.

Cornflower recipes

Cornflower eye bath or wash for sunburn

Ingredients / equipment
- » 1 tbsp dried cornflowers, or 2–3 tsp fresh ones – assume one to two loosely cupped hands full of the fresh, whole flowers
- » 300 ml (10 fl oz) boiling water
- » coffee filter paper

Instructions   Roughly chop the flowers if using fresh ones, and pile them into a jug or large mug, then pour over the boiling water. Let it infuse for 5–10 minutes, then strain through a coffee filter paper to make sure any tiny hairs or fibres have been removed. Once cooled, use as a bath to relieve eye strain or inflammation. This recipe can also be used as a skin wash, or a clean cloth soaked with the tea can be applied to ulcers, bites or blisters to bring relief.

Cornflower wound balm

Ingredients
- » 1 pint, loosely packed, of cornflowers and leaves
- » organic seed oil
- » lavender or Frankincense essential oil
- » 12 g beeswax for each 100 ml (3½ fl oz) oil

Instructions   As with all infused oils, shred the flowers and leaves and pack them into the double boiler top, then pour over enough oil to cover and infuse it for at least half an hour. Strain the resulting oil through a muslin or piece of kitchen towel and compost the remains of the spent herbs. To each 100 ml of oil add 12 g of beeswax and return both ingredients to the top of the double boiler. Warm until dissolved, add 5–10 drops of essential oil for each 100 ml of oil, then pour into clean, dry glass jars. Apply liberally to cuts, grazes, bites and stings to encourage healing.

Cornflower and limeflower sleep and nerve elixir

Ingredients
- » 1 pint each of fresh cornflowers and limeflowers
- » brandy or vodka, as preferred
- » local honey

Instructions　Pile the roughly chopped herbs into a large jar and pour over enough alcohol to just cover the plant matter, adding a couple of decent tablespoonfuls of local honey, before putting the lid on and giving it a good shake-up. Press the herbs under the alcohol again and let the whole lot sit for at least a fortnight, stirring every couple of days and pressing the herbs down again. After a few weeks, filter out the herbs and bottle the elixir. Take 5 ml (1 tsp) to ease anxiety, or 10 ml (2 tsp) through the course of the evening to encourage restful sleep.

Cornflower tonic

Very like the above recipe, this is a basic tonic that can be made with alcohol or vinegar. Just shred the herbs and pile into a glass jar, then pour over enough alcohol or vinegar to cover the plant matter. Put the lid on and shake it up every couple of days, leaving it to steep in a cool, dark cupboard until the herbs have thoroughly infused. Add spoonfuls of the vinegar to glasses of water, or use it neat on a cotton-wool pad to relieve bites and stings. The alcohol-based version can be taken on a daily basis as an all-round tonic – 5 ml (1 tsp) three times a day should suffice.

Elder
Sambucus nigra

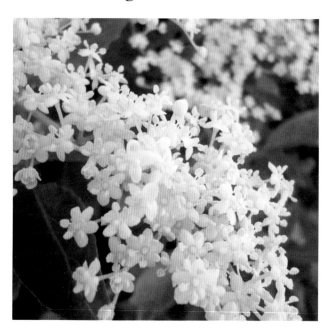

Also known as: devil's eye, lady elder, frau holle, tree of doom, old lady, lady ellhorn, whistle tree, pipe tree, black elder, bore tree, bour tree, hylder, hylantree, eldrum, ellhorn, Hollunder [German], sureau [French], the elder mother, the queen of herbs, old lady, old sal

Family Caprifoliaceae.

Habitat and description The elder tree is a familiar sight growing along roadsides, by paths and in hedgerows all across the UK. It tends to be more of a shrub than a tree, with pinnate leaves featuring serrated edges. The flowers form in wide, flat clusters and are creamy white in appearance, with five petals to each flower and a familiar, grape like fragrance. The berries are a rich purple-black and hang in heavy clusters known as drupes.

The bark of the tree is usually a pale brown-grey colour, often with rough grooves to the surface on the more mature trees. Elder is well known for its willingness to grow almost anywhere, from well-drained soil to stony soil or by the sea, but it particularly loves to grow near human habitation. The tree can grow up to 9m (30 ft) tall but doesn't usually grow much taller than this. When it is part of a hedgerow that gets trimmed regularly, I have noticed a marked tendency of the plant to grow upwards instead of outwards, with new shoots pointing very definitively skywards. The older twigs have a centre filled with white pith, which is easily removed – perhaps giving rise to many of its old names.

Where to find it   The UK and Europe, North America, many other temperate regions; Ireland, Asia. Mexico has a related plant used in much the same way.

Parts used   Commonly the flowers and fruit are used; less commonly, the leaves and bark.

When to gather   Young leaves and bark in March and April and flowers in June; berries from August onwards, as soon as they are deep purplish black and drooping downwards.

Medicines to make   Elderberry rob, syrup, elixir, wine or electuary; elderflower syrup, cordial, tea or wine for the immune system; leaves and bark in oil as an infused oil, salve or balm for bruises and bumps.

Constituents   The flowers contain triterpenes, including ursolic and oleanolic acid, as well as fixed oils containing free fatty acids, such as linolenic and palmitic acid; also flavonoids, including rutin, and other substances such as phenolic acids, as well as pectin and sugar. The leaves contain triterpenes similar to those in the flowers, as well as cyanogenetic glyco-sides and flavonoids such as rutin and quercitin.

Planetary influence   Venus.

Associated Deities   Hel, Hela, Holda, Hilde, dryads, Earth Goddesses with a distinct link to the Underworld, fairies, crone aspects of the Goddess such as Cailleach, Hecate, Cerridwen, The Morrigan, Lilith, Kali, etc.

Festival   Samhain.

Constitution   The whole plant is cool and neutral in temperament.

Actions and indications   Elder is a rich storehouse of medicines and properties, gaining it a well-earned reputation as the medicine chest of the people. The berries are a rich source of vitamin C, and the flowers combine well with yarrow (*Achillea*

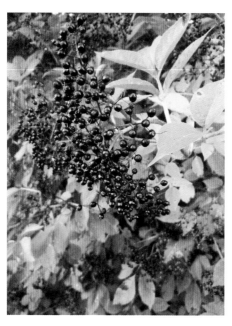

millefolium) and peppermint (*Mentha piperita*) as a cold and influenza remedy – two parts each of the yarrow and elderflower to one part of mint is the standard combination; 1 tsp of the dried mix can be infused in a cup of hot water and drunk three times a day. Elderflower can be used to relieve colds and influenza, chills, early stages of fevers and problems such as catarrh, sinusitis, tonsillitis and night sweats (this last if taken as a cold infusion). Unsurprisingly enough, given the history of usage for influenza, the flowers are a blood purifier, and the whole plant is antibacterial and antiviral. The flowers and berries can be combined with St John's wort as a potent antiviral, though this would need to be used with caution if you are on medication prescribed by your GP. The flowers can also be used at the onset of measles and chickenpox, as they bring out the rash and speed recovery. Use them externally to relieve itching and psoriasis, especially where this has formed blisters and pustules. The flowers also have an affinity with the kidneys and can relieve water retention and improve kidney function as a result.

Some are of the opinion that the juice of elderberries can be a useful remedy for long-standing rheumatism, neuralgia and sciatica.

The flowers as a whole reduce oedema of the mucous membranes in the nose and bronchi and can be combined with ground ivy and plantain as a useful remedy for hay fever and allergies. The leaves are emollient and vulnerary and make a superb ointment for the treatment of bruises, bumps, sprains, strains and chilblains. The bark of two-year-old twigs is purgative, vulnerary and anti-rheumatic; however, being violently purgative, it is not used internally. Externally, the bark can be used as an anti-rheumatic ointment or oil and combines really well with the young leaves for this purpose. You can also use a balm of this for bruises and bumps.

Folklore   Some consider the plant to have a slightly psycho-active effect, which is possibly the cause of at least some of the legends surrounding the tree.

The Romany gypsies call the tree *Yakori bengeskro*, or devil's eye, and forbid burning it. This is possibly at least partly because elder doesn't burn at all well, with the final deterrent being the legends surrounding the tree!

There are a number of theories surrounding the tree's name. One school of thought is that the name comes from the Anglo-Saxon *aeld*, meaning fire, possibly due to the fact that the twigs and smaller branches can be hollowed out and used to blow air into the base of the fire.

There is also a wide body of folklore surrounding Elda-Mor, the Elder Mother, also known as Hyldemoer in Scandinavian and Danish myth. This powerful spirit worked strong earth magic and would wreak revenge on any who harmed her host trees. A charm was crafted to be spoken before trying to take anything from the tree, running along the lines of 'Elder Mother, give me some of thy wood, and I'll give thee some of mine when I grow into a tree'. According to some sources, this charm originated in Lincolnshire, though I suspect variations can be found around the country. This charm was reputed to ward off harm that might arise from cutting the wood out of hand and without asking per-mission. The tree has a highly colourful reputation, being hailed by some as a benevolent forest spirit and by others as a vindictive demon, though I rather suspect this is merely a matter of personal perspective. Christian legend has it that Judas hanged himself from an elder tree after betraying Jesus, after which the elder ceased to achieve true tree status and instead dwindled into more of a shrub. Personally I think that as the elder tends to stand as a guardian between this world and other realms, shrub status suits this job rather better than being a huge tree that would find it hard to keep an eye on comings and goings!

There is a legend that babies should not be placed in cradles made of elder, or Hyldemoer would drag the child out by the ankles. This is possibly not too surprising, due to the elder tree's long-standing reputation as a tree of the Crone Goddess rather than the Maiden or Mother. Elder wood should not be made into house furniture either for similar reasons.

The tree is considered one of the ultimate trees of the White Goddess, due to the five petals on each flower. It is under the protection of the Old Crone aspect of the Goddess, and as a result is also associated with waning moon Goddesses. Throughout Europe the tree is associated with death and regeneration and magic – you can cut an elder right down to the base and she'll just regenerate. Interestingly, the tree is credited with working alongside witches as well as being used to remove the effects of curses and hexes cast by malevolent witches, perhaps representing the dual aspect of the Goddess in her form as Dark Mother.

Elder has the calm, wise energy of the grandmother or traditional Wise Woman and is a wonderful tree to call on when making tough decisions and needing to keep a cool head.

In addition to warding off evil spirits and forces, the elder was also used to ward off thunderbolts and plagues as well as to deflect lightning. The tree was regarded as a tree of Faerie: it was used both to ward off Faerie and prevent livestock from being 'hag-ridden', but it was also reputed to allow a person to see the courts of Faerie ride past on Midsummer day if they sat under the tree while it was in flower. It used to be planted next to bakehouses in order to prevent the devil from being folded in with the bread dough – incidentally, this is also apparently where the tradition of putting a cross in the top of the loaf before baking came from!

Dose   One tsp of the dried flowers to a cup of hot water drunk up to three times a day; of the elixir or tincture of the flowers and fruit, 10 ml (2 tsp) three times a day.

Contraindications   The berries can provoke nausea if too many are eaten, especially the green ones. As previously mentioned, the bark and leaves can be purgative and should not be used internally except under the direction of a trained herbalist.

Elder recipes

Elderflower cordial

Ingredients
- » at least 10 heads of fresh elderflowers – try to pick them when they have that lovely creamy pollen in the middle, as they have by far the best flavour at this time
- » 500 g (1 lb 1½ oz) of brown sugar
- » the zest and juice of one organic lemon
- » 570 ml (20 fl oz) of water

Instructions   There are two ways of making this recipe. The first method involves making up a sugar syrup by dissolving the sugar in the water with the lemon juice and zest, simmering it until it begins to thicken, and then pouring it over the clean flowers and allowing it to steep overnight. The following day, you can pour off the syrup. The drawback with this method is that the elderflower often has natural yeasts on it, which means that there's a good chance your finished syrup will begin to ferment! This method works well for syrup you intend to use very quickly, as there is less heat to destroy that delicate elder flavour.

Method two, which lasts a great deal longer, involves snipping the flowers off the main stems and putting them into a pan with the water, lemon juice and zest, then simmering it gently for 10 minutes, with a lid on the pan. Strain out the herbs and add the sugar, returning to a gentle simmer until it has dissolved, then turn up the heat and boil it gently until it begins to thicken. This one may not have quite the same flavour as the first, but it lasts a lot longer as the yeast has been denatured by boiling it. Alternatively you can pour the water over the flowers and leave overnight, then strain out the elder and boil up the resulting liquid with the sugar and lemon juice to thicken it. I have tried all three methods, and all give tasty results. Some old recipes even call for citric acid, but I haven't found that necessary.

You could also do a version with fresh lemon balm from the garden as well as the elder – this makes a delicious cordial as well as an excellent country wine.

Elderflower and honeysuckle elixir

Ingredients
- » at least 10 heads of fresh elderflower
- » at least 1 pint of fresh honeysuckle flowers – you can add these later if need be
- » local honey
- » brandy

Instructions Check over the elder and snip the flowers into a Kilner jar, then add at least two large tablespoonfuls of honey and enough brandy to cover the flowers plus 2.5 cm (1 in.) extra on top. Put the lid on and allow this to steep for at least a fortnight – if you have honeysuckle flowers available immediately, you can put these in at the same time, or strain out the elderflower and add the honeysuckle later on.

This elixir is delicious and full of vitamin C, brilliant for summer colds, and also helpful in stress headaches made worse by heat. Definitely one for the store cupboard!

Elderflower tea

This tea is very simple to make and is wonderful for the relief of a summer cold, to encourage the body to sweat out a fever. Just pour the equivalent of one cup of hot water, just off the boil, over 1 tsp, heaped, of fresh or dried flowers, pop a plate over the top, and allow it to steep for 5 minutes. Sweeten with a little honey and drink it as hot as you can stand in order to bring on a good sweat.

If you would like to dry your elderflower, you need either a large table covered with greaseproof paper or large baskets – whichever is easiest and most convenient for you. Check the flowers for livestock and lay them out in the baskets or on the paper, making sure they do not touch each other. Leave them to dry for at least a week, turning them over every couple of days. The smell of drying elderflower can only be compared to that of cat wee, though it does improve as it dries – once you have rubbed all the flowers off the stems and put them into a jar, it will smell pleasant again, I promise! To remove the flowers from the stems once dry, just rub vigorously in circles between the palms, holding them over a large bowl. The flowers should drop free very easily, leaving the central stems to be composted.

Elderberry syrup

Ingredients
- » at least 10 heads of ripe elderberries
- » 1140 ml (40 fl oz) of water

» at least 1 kg (2 lb 3½ oz) of unrefined brown sugar
» 1 large organic lemon, or 2 smaller ones
» 1 stick of cinnamon, or 1 tsp, heaped, of ground cinnamon
» 5 cm (2 in.) piece of fresh root ginger
» 2 whole star anise, roughly ground

Instructions   Using either a fork or your fingertips, remove the elderberries from their stems. This is done as too much of the stalks and green berries can give you rather a bad stomach, so while you are removing the berries, try to take out as many green ones as you can. A few stray ones will do you no harm at all, just try not to allow too many to get in.

Put the berries into a large pan and pour over the water, then add the finely diced ginger, the cinnamon and star anise. Zest and juice the lemon and add this as well, then bring the whole lot to a gentle simmer. Allow the pan full of ingredients to simmer for at least 10 minutes – more like half an hour, if possible – to really pull the most flavour and goodness out of the berries and spices.

Once this is done, strain out all the ingredients and pour the liquid back into the pan, along with the sugar. I tend to allow 500 g (1 lb 1½ oz) of sugar to 570 ml (20 fl oz) of liquid, though you may want to add more if you would like it to keep for longer. Unfortunately the sugar is a major preservative in this recipe, so you do need to add plenty! Put the pan back onto a gentle heat for 10 minutes, until the sugar has dissolved, then bring to a boil and, stirring regularly, simmer until the liquid has thickened somewhat. Keep an eye on your syrup – any liquid with a high sugar content can burn very easily.

Once it has thickened a little, take the syrup off the heat and pour it into clean bottles, putting the lid on as soon as possible. Label your syrup with the date as well as the contents and store it in a dark, cool place, or in the fridge. Take 15–30 ml

(1–2 tbsp) daily as a prophylactic against coughs, colds and fever, or pour it over ice-cream or cakes or pudding, or stir it into hot water as a steaming hot drink after a cool afternoon.

Elderberry rob

Ingredients

- » as many bunches of elderberries as you can manage – I use at least 20, more if possible
- » star anise – I use two, but you can use more if you prefer it

Instructions   As with the recipe for the syrup above, remove all the berries from the stems, looking to keep out as many of the green ones as you can. Put the berries into a large pan with 50 ml (1¾ fl oz) of water, no more than that if possible, then put the whole thing onto a gentle heat with the roughly broken star anise, stirring occasionally until the berries begin to break and release their juices. Simmer the berries gently for at least half an hour, until all the berries have burst, then cool down until it is a temperature you are comfortable handling. Next comes the fun part – push the whole lot through a jelly bag or a large square of muslin. Expect to get very purple hands while doing this! You can wear rubber gloves if you want, but I reckon purple hands is something every herbalist should experience at least once!

Once you have squeezed out as much juice as you possibly can, you should find yourself with a scant few tablespoons of stones and fruit pulp, which you can put in the compost bin. Return the liquid to the pan, making sure there are no stones left sticking to the side of it, and put the whole thing back onto a gentle heat, allowing it to simmer for at least half an hour. What you are looking to do with this recipe is to allow as much water content to evaporate off as possible, which should leave you with a thick liquid in the bottom of the pan.

Once it has reduced as much as you want it to, scrape it quickly into a jar and allow it to cool, which should make it set almost solid. Make sure you use a jar for this, preferably one you can get a teaspoon or egg spoon into, as the rob will set completely, and if you have poured it into a bottle, you will be hard pressed to get it out again! Alternatively if you prefer, you can reduce it down just enough to make a thick liquid, which will not keep for quite as long but is every bit as effective as the paste version.

This recipe is a good deal more suitable for diabetics, as there is no added sugar, making it a lot kinder to the body.

Allow one small piece the size of a pea per day as a prophylactic, or stir it into fruit teas with a generous dollop of honey.

Elderberry and blackberry honey

Ingredients
- » at least 10 bunches of fresh elderberries
- » approximately ½ pint of fresh blackberries – you can use some from the freezer if you need to
- » one large jar of local runny honey

Instructions Remove the berries from the stems, as detailed in previous recipes. Put the blackberries into a pan with 50 ml (1¾ fl oz) of water. Bring the whole lot to a gentle simmer and keep stirring and mashing occasionally until all the berries have burst and released their juices, then take the pan off the heat.

Push the berries through a sieve to remove any small stones, then reduce down in the pan by around one third. Allow the pulp to cool to just above room temperature. Stir in the entire contents of the jar of honey, making sure it is all well folded together, then decant the resulting syrup back into jars, labelling it carefully. If you like a little more kick with this, you can add the juice and zest of a large lemon and a very finely diced piece of fresh root ginger, though this combination of flavours will be more suited to adults than children. This recipe lasts for at least six months, even if stored in the cupboard instead of the fridge.

Take 5 ml (1 tsp) a day as a prophylactic, or every couple of hours at the onset of a cold to help the body fight it off as quickly as possible.

Elder bud salve

Ingredients
- » at least ½ pint of loosely packed buds
- » organic seed oil
- » beeswax
- » essential oils; I like mint and rosemary for this recipe

Instructions   When you gather your buds, try not to take too many from a single tree, and restrict yourself to no more than two buds per branch if possible. Remember that the ideal is to not be able to see where you have foraged afterwards – too much is damaging to the tree and will reduce the amount of flowers and berries for you to gather later on. Make sure the buds are dry, with no water trapped within the new leaf folds, and finely chop them using a sharp knife, mezzaluna or food processor. Pack them into the top of a double boiler and just cover them with the seed oil, then fill the base with a little water and put the whole thing on to warm.

Let the herbs steep in the warming oil for at least half an hour, until the colour changes, then strain out the herbs. Allow 10–12 g beeswax per 100 ml (3½ fl oz) oil, and pop both ingredients back into the double boiler. Let it warm through and stir in 5 drops of each of your chosen essential oil – up to a maximum of 20 drops per 100 ml – and stir briefly before pouring the salve into small jars and putting the lids on. You can apply this salve to bruises, bumps, strains and sprains, sore muscles and arthritic joints, to relieve discomfort, dispel swelling and bruising and improve blood flow to the area.

Fumitory
Fumaria officinalis

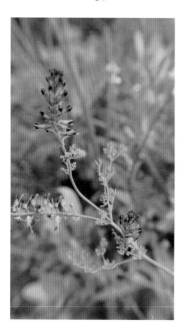

Also known as: earth smoke, wax dolls, kapnos, nidor, vapour, smoke-plant, lady's lockets, beggart, fumus

Family Fumariaceae.

Habitat and description This ethereal and beautiful annual can be found scrambling merrily through hedgerows and waste ground, where it will quite happily self-sow, but you will rarely find it growing in the same place two years in a row. Like smoke itself, fumitory goes where it will, and this free-spirited plant is very difficult indeed to actually cultivate. All you can really do is scatter the seed in a forgotten corner and hope the plant shows up to say hello.

Long, slender stems that are a silvery green colour play host to flower heads of pale pink and mauve, with touches of silvery green. The plant flowers between April and October, before setting seed and moving on. The leaves are deeply divided into lance-shaped lobes and a silvery green in colour, and the whole plant is delicate in appearance, looking very much, when seen at a distance, as though it is smoke that has emerged from the earth.

Where to find it   Parts of Europe; the UK and Ireland; temperate regions of North Africa and Asia; parts of North America, though it is not much used there.

Parts used   The whole flowering tops.

When to gather   When the plant is in flower, throughout the summer.

Medicines to make   Decoctions, juices, infusions and tinctures; teas and washes; pills and powders.

Constituents   The plant contains a range of alkaloids, including fumaricine, fumariline and fumaritine, as well as the antiseptic sanguinarine; hydroxycinnamic acid derivatives; and fumaric acid, caffeic and chlorogenic acid, flavonoids, bitter components, plus mucilage.

Planetary influence   Saturn.

Associated deities and heroes   None specific, but given the herb's association with the Underworld, most likely linked to Earth and Underworld deities.

Constitution   Cool and moist.

Actions and indications   Fumitory is used as a short-term tonic, with gentle diuretic and laxative properties. It has been used to relieve stomach disorders stemming from improper levels of digestive enzymes being produced and released, as well as acting as an overall tonic for sluggish liver function – consider combining it with meadowsweet and dandelion root for these sorts of issues.

It is painkilling and antispasmodic to the whole digestive tract, especially to the stomach and liver, and is amphoteric, or normalising, to biliary flow. It can be used for impaired function of the gall bladder and liver, with the attendant issues of pain, exhaustion, nausea, bloating, headaches and fat intolerance that go with it, making it ideal for treating fatty liver disorder as well as other hepatic issues where flow of bile is impaired or reduced.

As it is antispasmodic and gently painkilling, it can be used to relieve gallstones and gallstone pain, and its liver stimulant and tonic properties mean that it can be very helpful in relieving constipation. It is considered an excellent blood cleanser and alterative, used in the treatment of chronic eczema and psoriasis, especially where this is due to the liver not functioning at its most optimum – by extension, I also recommend it as a short-term assistant to encourage better metabolism

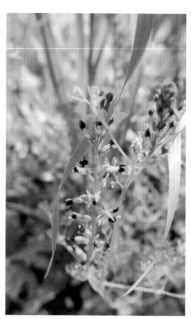

of hormones out of the body, therefore helping with acne related to menstruation. It has an old reputation for boosting thyroid function and improving sluggish metabolism – it will literally teach you the lessons of air and movement instead of being static and stuck.

Its close relative, Indian fumitory, is hepatoprotective, so there is a fair chance the British version can be used for this as well, especially when you take into account all the other really useful affinities the British version has with the liver, gall bladder and pancreas.

Its alterative properties also make it helpful for the relief of rheumatic disorders, acting as a blood cleanser. It boasts some gentle diuretic properties that help with the all-round removal of toxins from the system, and can also be used to gently lower the blood pressure.

A tea of the herb can be used to help the body to eliminate intestinal parasites.

Topically it can be used to make salves and washes to heal wounds and rashes – a compress of the juice can be very helpful here – and in addition to this, for the treatment of stubborn eczema and psoriasis. It is recommended to take the herb internally as well as externally, and remember that when treating skin issues, there is often a healing crisis before the situation begins to resolve itself.

Folklore   It is thought that fumitory resembles vapour leaving the earth, hence its name, earth smoke. It was ranked as a weed in Galen's time, as it will gladly get its roots into the ground in fields and verges, becoming difficult to eradicate as a result. It is far more commonly found in the east of the country than further west.

Dose   Tea made with 1 tsp of the dried herb to a cup of water three times a day, or up to 1 ml twice a day of the tincture. Fumitory doesn't store well dried, and its medicinal properties deteriorate quickly, like smoke drifting away on the wind. If you can juice it and store the juice, that works well, or tincture it fresh where possible.

Contraindications   Large doses have a laxative effect. Taken over long periods of time, the plant can become very addictive, so it is best to use it two weeks on, one week off to avoid building up a tolerance to it. Not advised for use by pregnant women.

Fumitory recipes

Liver tonic blend for fatty liver

Ingredients
- » 2–3 handfuls of fresh fumitory herb
- » dried dandelion root (if you have any)
- » ground milk thistle seeds (if you have any)
- » vodka or brandy

Instructions   Grind up or bruise the seeds and dandelion root if you have them, then shred or finely chop the fumitory and pile it into a clean glass jar, pouring over the alcohol until covered, with 2.5 cm (1 in.) extra on top. Give it a quick stir to make sure the herbs have soaked up all the alcohol, then put the lid on, and store it in a dark cupboard, shaking or stirring it up every other day. If you don't have the dried dandelion root and milk thistle seeds, don't worry – you can always add fresh chopped dandelion root in the autumn, and repeat the process. If just using fumitory on its own, let the herbs and alcohol steep for at least two weeks, then strain out the herbs, and bottle the alcohol. Take 1 ml twice a day for two weeks, then take at least a week off – a pipette with millilitre markings up the side can be really useful here!

Fumitory compress for eczema and psoriasis

All you need here is several decent handfuls of the herb, checked to ensure cleanliness. It really doesn't matter if the herbs are wet when being gathered, as the idea here is to create a compress, not to dry them. Finely chop the herbs using a sharp knife or herb chopper, or even a food processor, and mix a tiny bit of warm water with it to create a thick paste – start off adding a teaspoon at a time, until the herbs clump together easily. Smear a thick layer of the chopped herbs onto a large square of muslin or a piece of clean tea towel, then apply it to the area affected with eczema or psoriasis, leaving it for at least 10 minutes to really soak. Wrap it with a bit of cling film to hold it in place if possible – don't leave the poultice on for too long though, as both of these skin conditions need to breathe! If the skin problems are in awkward places, like behind the ears, squeeze out as much juice from the poultice as you can and apply the juice to the area using a cotton-wool pad or a clean cloth that can be washed afterwards. Do this a couple of times a day if possible.

Fumitory and meadowsweet acid balancer for the digestive tract

Ingredients
 » ½ pint each of fumitory and meadowsweet leaves and flowering tops
 » vodka (optional)

Instructions   This can be made in two different ways: either dry the herbs, thoroughly chop them, and use them as a tea, which will better suit those with peptic ulceration, or wilt the herbs for a few days, thoroughly chop them, and turn them into a cottage tincture blend by piling them into a jar, pouring over plenty of vodka and letting them steep for a few weeks before straining the herbs out. Take one dropperful in a glass of water up to three times a day for no more than a week, to encourage stomach acid levels to normalise.

Honeysuckle
Lonicera periclymenum

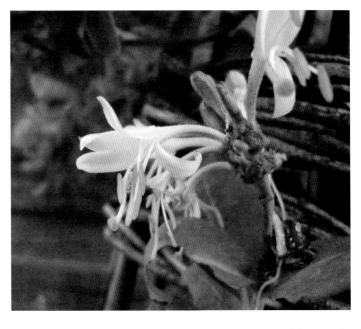

Also known as: woodbine, goat leaf, mother of the woods, evening pride, fairy trumpets

Family   Caprifoliaceae.

Habitat and description   A popular garden plant, honeysuckle can also be found growing in woodlands and scrambling merrily up country hedges and train-track banks, preferring to grow in light shade where possible. It is a fast-growing climber with roughly ovate leaves in opposite pairs that have a slightly waxy finish to them, meaning that rain droplets look rather silvery on them.

The flowers are quite long and slender, with extravagantly trumpet-shaped openings, and usually warm golden yellow, often with a pink tone to them, especially as they age. They are strongly scented and much beloved of both bees and humans. The plant is a woody perennial that can grow to heights of 6 m (20 ft), given a tree tall enough – I used to have them outside a second-story bedroom window, where they would flower with great abandon, but not at all closer to ground. The flowers are followed by poisonous red berries in the autumn.

Where to find it   Found commonly throughout the UK and Ireland, and in most other temperate regions of the world, including most of Europe, North Africa and South West Asia.

Parts used   Flowers (some herbalists also use the leaves and occasionally the berries, but I stick to just the flowers).

When to gather   June through to September.

Medicines to make   Honeysuckle tea, elixir and tincture for coughs and colds; honeysuckle skin wash; honeysuckle-infused oil or salve for chilblains and insect bites and stings; honeysuckle vinegar for sunburn.

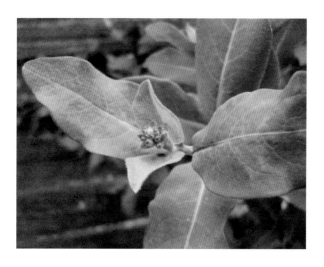

Constituents   Saponins and loganic acid, according to some sources, but very little research has been done into the components of the honeysuckle. It is highly likely that it contains iridoids and essential oils as well as flavones, based on the constituents in its relative, *Lonicera japonica*. The English version is also rich in salicylic acid, making it a great painkiller and anti-inflammatory.

Planetary influence   Jupiter.

Associated deities and heroes   Cerridwen, all faery queens, Pan.

Festival   Midsummer.

Constitution   Cold and moist.

Actions and indications   Honeysuckle seems to have sadly fallen out of use in the UK, which is a real shame, given its many indications and uses. American herbalists use it for coughs and colds as a vitamin-C-rich tonic, and also for headaches linked with heat. I have certainly found it very helpful for this, as well as for headaches from a sudden rise in body temperature due to stress or anger. It has been used as an expectorant, to help the body rid itself of unnecessary phlegm, and also as a cooling laxative for overheated systems.

As an extension of the cooling properties, any other 'hot' conditions – hot flashes during the menopause, hot, inflamed joints, hot tempers and anxiety causing sleeplessness – may well benefit from honeysuckle. The presence of salicylic acid makes it anti-inflammatory and painkilling as well as cooling: ideal in the treatment of any inflamed conditions ranging from sore throat to arthritis. It also has a historical reputation as being a liver and spleen herb, though it is not much used for that these days, as far as I can tell. It is, however, a lovely nervine, which I have noticed from personal experience – although, again from personal experience, it doesn't suit anyone with a cold constitution, as it is simply too cooling. In brief: those with anxiety and insomnia may get on very well with this herb, whereas it may not suit those prone to depression too well.

Externally, it can be used to make a wonderful cooling and soothing skin wash for sunburn, eczema, insect bites and stings and other itchy skin issues, as well as to make an infused oil for chilblains, rheumatism and arthritis, especially where redness and heat can be seen around the joint.

Japanese honeysuckle is still used widely in Chinese medicine, to reduce heat in the body and cool the blood, and from what I have seen, these properties equally apply to our native honeysuckle.

Folklore   Honeysuckle is linked with love and devotion in the language of flowers, and, grown in the garden, it brings prosperity and protection from evil. If it is growing around the door, it brings good luck to the household.

Dose   Five ml (1 tsp) of the elixir, 2.5 ml (½ tsp) of the tincture, made cottage-style, up to three times a day (more often than this will cause nausea); 1 tsp, heaped, of the dried flowers infused in a cup of water twice a day, or roughly 10 fresh flowers (individual ones, not flower heads) infused in hot water twice a day.

Contraindications   High doses can cause nausea and vomiting.

Honeysuckle recipes

Honeysuckle and lemon balm honey

Ingredients

- » large handfuls each of fresh honeysuckle flowers and fresh lemon balm leaves
- » a large jar of local honey – if you can get limeflower or linden honey, so much the better

Instructions   This recipe is delightfully simple to make! Just slowly immerse your clean, pest-free honeysuckle flowers in the honey, stirring gently to get them to sink downwards. Check the lemon balm for insects or dirt and chop it finely, then do the same with them. Cover the pot with a sheet of kitchen roll or a square of muslin held in place with a rubber band, and pop the jar on a sunny windowsill, stirring occasionally to push the flowers under the level of the honey again. Once a fortnight has passed, strain the lot through a sieve to remove the flowers. If need be, stand the jar in a bowl of warm water first to encourage it into an even more runny form that will go through the sieve easily.

Take 5 ml (1 tsp) to calm the mood and ease stress, or use it to sweeten a cup of lemon balm, chamomile, limeflower or other soothing tea.

Honeysuckle and elderberry elixir

Ingredients
  » fresh honeysuckle flowers
  » fresh elderberries – at least half a dozen large bunches
  » brandy, or whichever spirit is your preference
  » local honey
  » fresh root ginger – 5 cm (2 in.) piece
  » star anise – two entire stars

Instructions   Using your fingers, remove the elderberries from their stems and cook very gently with 15 ml (1 tbsp) water until all the juices have been extracted from the berries; take off the heat and squeeze out through a clean jelly cloth, glorying in the purple fingers you will gain as you do. Pour the resulting liquid into a large Kilner jar and add several handfuls of fresh honeysuckle flowers – you can add these on a day-to-day basis if you need to, as unless you have access to a particularly large honeysuckle plant, getting enough flowers in one go may be problematic.

Finely shred the ginger root and put that into the Kilner jar, along with the roughly crushed star anise and at least three large tablespoons of local honey, then pour over approximately double to triple the amount of brandy as you have added elderberry juice. Put the lid on and shake it up thoroughly to get it all to mix together, then put it into a cool, dark cupboard for at least a fortnight. You can keep adding honeysuckle flowers periodically and shaking it back up again to get it all to mix together.

After a good fortnight or two, strain out the herbs and spices and pour the resulting elixir into bottles. Label it clearly and take 10 ml (2 tsp) in the evening as a cough, cold and flu prophylactic, or take 10 ml up to three times a day if you already have the beginnings of a cold. Stirring it into a cup of hot water with lemon and ginger can be a lovely way to relieve the symptoms of a cold.

Honeysuckle and rose sunburn spray

Ingredients
- » plenty of fresh honeysuckle flowers
- » plenty of fresh rose petals – *Rosa gallica* or *damascena* is best, if you can find it, but any fragranced old English rose will work well
- » white wine or cider vinegar
- » aromatic water – lavender or rose is superb; if this is hard to get hold of, a tea of lavender flowers can be used instead

Instructions   Pack the flowers into a jar and pour over plenty of the vinegar – don't be afraid to keep adding handfuls of flowers as they open, as if you only have a small amount available at any given time it can be hard to gather enough for the recipe in one go. If you need to top up the vinegar with every few handfuls of herbs added, then do this. Let the whole lot steep for at least two weeks, then strain out the herbs and dilute with an equal amount of aromatic water or lavender tea. Pour the resulting mixture into a spray bottle and use it on sunburn, insect bites and stings, to soothe redness and take the heat out of these troublesome issues. With sunburn, follow it up with a moisturising cream of rose or lavender once the heat has gone out of the affected area.

Knapweed – Black / Greater
Centaurea nigra / Centaurea scabiosa

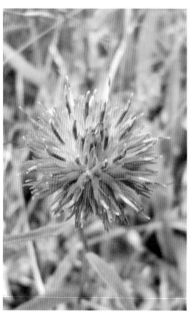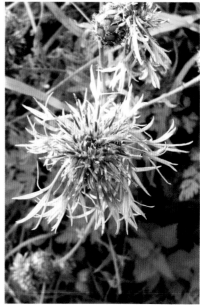

Also known as: hardheads, star thistle, ironweed, bullweed, logger head, boltsede, matt felon, hard irons

Family Asteraceae.

Habitat and description This perennial denizen of hedgerows and meadows has a basal rosette of leaves in the spring; these are a silvery green in colour, toothed and divided, and rising into tough stems with globular flower heads, part of which in *Centaurea nigra* are black on the outer scales, giving rise to the Latin name of *nigra*, or 'black'. The flowers themselves are a rich mauve-purple colour and bloom in profusion – much beloved by bees, they are also frequented by moths and other insects, which rely on them as a valuable nectar plant throughout the summer. The whole plant grows to up to 1 m (3 ft) tall and can form quite bushy clumps, given enough room to thrive.

Where to find it   Native to the UK and Europe but has naturalised in other temperate regions, where it is sometimes considered a problem plant.

Parts used   Aerial parts and roots.

When to gather   Summer, once the plant is in flower. For the roots, wait until autumn, when the plant has gone dormant.

Medicines to make   Decoctions for sore throats, poor digestion and over-relaxed mucous membranes; infused oils, salves, balms and poultices for wounds and inflamed glands; a tincture of the whole plant for long-term storage, and also as a spray for cuts and grazes.

Constituents   Flavonoids.

Planetary influence   Saturn.

Associated deities and heroes   Linked with Chiron and Hercules.

Constitution   Cool and dry.

Actions and indications   Historically used for bleeding and sore throats, knapweed has rather fallen out of common usage these days, but it does have a few uses that are worth mentioning. Generally, knapweed is used externally for wound healing, for which it has a powerful affinity – use it for haemorrhoids and piles, varicose veins and spider veins as a double-infused salve, or for bruising, wounds and ruptures. It has a long history of use for whitlows, or inflamed fingernails – there's that astringent property coming into good use again.

Internally, it has been used as a digestive tonic, to soothe inflamed mucous membranes and to encourage healthier digestive function. It has some possible antiviral properties as well, making it potentially a good addition to remedies to beat viral infections, such as shingles. No noted effect on the liver has been found, so it is entirely possible that this would make a useful remedy for those unable to use St John's wort.

Like many plants ruled by Saturn, this herb is concerned with restoring borders and boundaries to the body. As an astringent, it can be used to reduce excess mucus in the lungs and stomach and would combine well with ground ivy and plantain for this purpose as a handy remedy for mopping up after the common cold.

A strong decoction of the leaves and flowering tops is, in spite of its astringent properties, a useful and gentle diuretic and can be used to strengthen the kidneys.

The flowers are edible and can be added to salads and other recipes, and the plant itself is a wonderful land healer – restoring good health to poor soil and dying back once this process is complete.

Folklore   Legend has it that the famed centaur healer Chiron discovered the virtues of this herb by using it to cure a wound caused by the profligate use of poisoned arrows by Hercules. Ever since, the plant has been used to treat deep wounds and bruises and was even tried as a Plague cure.

Much like the humble daisy, knapweed blooms were used for the well-known 'loves me, loves me not' charm, as young girls would pick off the petals and chant the rhyme to divine whether the object of their interests returned their favour. Another piece of folklore reckons that unmarried girls would wear the flower buds in their bodice – they would bloom if they stumbled across their future partner.

Dose   Little is known about correct dosage for this plant; however a standard one could be 5 ml (1 tsp) of the chopped herb to a cup of hot water, infused and drunk three times a day. If you are using a cottage tincture, assume 2.5–5 ml (½–1 tsp) up to three times a day.

Contraindications   None known at present.

Knapweed recipes

Scabious (*Knautia arvensis*) [field scabious, bachelor's buttons] is not related but can be used in the same way.

Knapweed decoction for sore throats

Ingredients
  » 1 pint of roughly chopped knapweed aerial parts, or quarter of a pint of roughly chopped root
  » 570 ml (20 fl oz) of water

Instructions   Pile the chopped ingredients into a saucepan and cover with the water, then bring to a simmer for at least half an hour. Aim for the water content to have reduced by at least half. Strain out the herbs, cool to a comfortable temperature, and drink in half-cup doses. If gargling with it, gargle with quarter of the cup, spitting out half of it and swallowing the other half.

Knapweed double-infused balm for wounds

Ingredients
  » 2 lots of 1 pint of knapweed flowering tops and leaves
  » organic seed oil
  » beeswax

Instructions   Thoroughly chop the plants, a job that may be easier using kitchen scissors, as those stems are tough. Pile the chopped herbs into a double boiler and cover with the oil, then leave to infuse over a gentle heat for at least an hour. Filter out the first lot of herbs and repeat the process with the second batch, then leave to cool. Filter out the spent herbs and compost them, then measure out the oil. To each

100 ml (3½ fl oz) of the oil add 12 g of beeswax, and add both ingredients back to the double boiler. Warm and stir until the beeswax has melted, then pour it into jars. You can add essential oils for fragrance if you prefer – go for healing scents if possible, such as lavender, chamomile, frankincense or myrrh. This balm can be used on all sorts of cuts, grazes, bruises, varicose veins or piles.

Knapweed, nettle and ground ivy tonic for after colds

Ingredients
  - » 2 handfuls each of fresh nettle, knapweed flowering tops and ground ivy
  - » vodka or brandy
  - » local honey

Instructions   This is another of the elixir blends that will need making throughout the year: either separate elixirs of each plant (which I highly recommend – that way you are getting four medicines for your work instead of just one) or, if space is at a premium, simply one large jar to which you add each ingredient as it comes into season, beginning with nettle tops in the spring, adding ground ivy later on, and finishing up with the knapweed. Don't forget to add honey or maple syrup if you want to sweeten the taste. Make sure the herbs are well covered with alcohol – if you are using the one-pot method, you may need to add more alcohol each time you add the fresh lot of herbs. Shake the mixture up every couple of days. Steep until two weeks after the last lot of herbs has gone in, then strain out the herbs and bottle the liquid. Take 5 ml (1 tsp) up to four times a day to help the body expel excess mucus, dry up post-nasal drip and settle mucus production back down to normal.

Lady's mantle
Alchemilla vulgaris / Alchemilla mollis

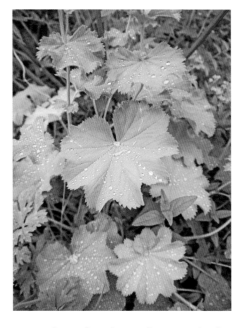

Also known as: lion's foot, bear's foot, nine hooks,
leontopodium, stellaria, dewcup, a woman's best friend,
nine monks, breakstone, piercestone, fair with tears, water carrier,
water chalice flower, ever-dew, mary's mantle, great sanicle

Family   Rosaceae.

Habitat and description   The lovely lady's mantle is a truly
delightful perennial, with large roughly kidney-shaped leaves
that have lightly toothed edges and are covered in a very light
downy hair, more so on *Alchemilla mollis* than on the wild
version *A. vulgaris*, though both can be used in much the

same way. The plant was believed by the alchemists of old to have great power – hence the Latin name *Alchemilla*, or little alchemist. It has the delightful habit of collecting liquid in the centre and around the edges of her leaves first thing in the morning – droplets of water that shimmer like a crystal out of a fairy tale. The "dew" is actually water that the plant exudes. This pretty plant is fairly low-growing and easy-going, as long as she has a reasonable amount of sun – and will reward you with many leaves, brilliant, filmy yellow-green flowers, with a tendency to self-seed.

Lady's mantle has masses of tiny pale-green flowers in summer, and although some authors decry these flowers as being rather insignificant, if you look closely they are as lacy as filigree and resemble a fine mist in large enough quantities, adding a charmingly fragile air to the herb garden. Personally, I love the whole plant, from the leaf and its dewdrops to the tiny greenish-yellow flowers. The plant usually doesn't grow much taller than 30 cm (1 ft) high and dies back during the winter, sprouting new, gloriously blue-green leaves in the spring. Look at your plant several times a week to truly appreciate the new leaves slowly unfurling into their typical cloak shape.

Where to find it   Most cool temperate regions, including the UK and Europe, parts of Scandinavia, Asia, North America and Africa. The range of different members of this plant family is quite wide.

Parts used   Leaves and flowers, also occasionally the fresh root.

When to gather   From mid-spring through to late summer, particularly when the plant flowers from June onwards.

Constituents   Tannins; tannic glycosides; bitters, salicylic acid; flavonoids; saponins.

Planetary influence   Venus.

Associated deities and heroes   Generally sacred to Earth Goddesses; the Virgin Mary; Mother Goddesses.

Constitution   Moderate and dry.

Actions and indications   Given the plant's common name, it should come as no great surprise to learn that the herb is predominantly used for many of the problems and imbalances associated with the female reproductive system. As a uterine tonic, it can be used to relieve painful periods and cramping, as well as to improve fertility in general, for which it is particularly well suited to women over 35 who are trying to conceive, though I would also be inclined to combine it with raspberry leaf and give it to all women who want a healthy pregnancy – be sure that the woman is not already pregnant first, though, just in case, as both of these herbs can cause cramping. Different herbalists have varying opinions on the safety of these herbs, but in the early stages of pregnancy it pays to be safe rather than sorry.

Some give it to pregnant women who are bleeding a little and fear a miscarriage, though only in small amounts, as larger amounts can bring on labour. It can also be used to encourage contractions during labour, when things are progressing too slowly. After birth it can be given to women who are bleeding excessively, in order to stop post-partum haemorrhage. Because it is a uterine tonic, it will help the womb to return to its normal size and healthy tone after pregnancy and birth, as well as acting to heal the uterus after abortion or miscarriage. It can also be given to women who have fibroids or pelvic inflammatory disease, especially where this is causing heavy bleeding.

During the menopause, lady's mantle can reduce excessive bleeding and ease the accompanying sweating. It can be used to relieve hormone-related anxiety causing PMS and menopausal anxiety.

Used topically and internally, the herb speeds the healing of wounds, and, when applied as a lotion or wash, it encourages the drying of a wound, bringing the edges together and encouraging healing. Add to a bath after childbirth to speed the healing of perineal tears.

Applied as an infused oil as well as drunk in tea form, the herb is reputed to restore tone and elasticity to breast tissue. It can be applied as a leaf compress soaked in a tea made from more of the leaves, for the same purpose.

Because the plant is astringent, it can be used for some cases of diarrhoea, especially when this is related to atony of the intestines. In addition to this, it can prove useful for those who struggle with nausea after eating fatty foods.

Folklore   The plant was originally associated with the Virgin Mary – hence the common name of the plant, as the leaves are supposed to resemble a woman's mantle or cloak.

The Latin name apparently derives from the Arabic word *alkemelych*, meaning alchemy, which was given to the plant due to its many virtues. The alchemists used to add the dewdrops collected on the plant's leaves to their mixtures, as they believed that the water had strong magical powers.

Dose   Five ml (1 tsp) per cup of hot water, drunk three times a day, or as required. No more than 15 ml (1 tbsp) of the tincture as a single dose – and I would suggest this as suitable only when you need to stop heavy bleeding or diarrhoea. For a more tonic effect, use smaller quantities on a daily basis – many herbalists recommend 2–4 ml three times a day.

Contraindications   According to some, it should not be used during pregnancy; others express no such caution and actually recommend it as a partus preparator before birth. Personally, I think it is best to be safe rather than sorry.

Lady's mantle recipes

A tonic elixir for uterine health

Ingredients
- » ½ pint of each of the following herbs, moderately packed:
  - – raspberry leaf
  - – rose petals
  - – lady's mantle leaves
  - – lemon balm
- » brandy or vodka
- » honey

Instructions If you are using fresh herbs, finely chop the ingredients and pile them into a Kilner jar. Dried herbs can be used as is – assume 2 tbsp of each herb. Add a couple of large tablespoonfuls of the honey, then pour over plenty of brandy to cover the herbs. Stir it thoroughly, put the lid on and leave it to steep for at least a fortnight, shaking occasionally. After this time, strain out the herbs and put the elixir into a storage bottle – ideally one with a dropper. Take 5 ml (1 tsp) twice a day as a general uterine tonic, and drops as needed to help recover physically and emotionally from miscarriage or abortion.

Lady's mantle wash for wounds and tears

Ingredients
- » ½ pint of fresh leaves
- » 570 ml (20 fl oz) of hot water just off the boil

Instructions Finely chop the herbs and pile them into a bowl or jug, then pour over the water and stir briefly. Leave the whole lot to cool and infuse as it does so, then strain out the herbs. Use as a wash for cuts and grazes, or to bathe perineal tears after birth, to encourage healing.

Lady's mantle and rose cream for breast care

Ingredients
- » fresh lady's mantle leaves
- » fresh rose petals (if you have any – if not, use dried ones, plus essential oils)
- » organic sunflower oil
- » vegetable glycerine
- » vitamin E oil or rosehip seed oil
- » flower waters, or strong tea of rose or lady's mantle
- » beeswax
- » rose essential oil

Instructions   Gather the lady's mantle on a dry day and finely chop it, then pile it into a double boiler, cover with oil, and infuse for at least half an hour. For an extra strong cream, double infuse the leaves by filtering out the first lot and repeating the process with fresh plant matter. If you are using rose petals, add these in with the leaves, adding up to equal amounts of petals to leaves. Once the oil is as strong as you want it to be, strain out the herbs through muslin or kitchen roll, and let the oil settle to ensure that it is clear. Allow 8–10 g of beeswax per 100 ml (3½ fl oz) of oil, and put the two ingredients back into the double boiler – add the rosehip seed oil at this point if you are using it, but remember to include it in the calculated total amount of oil. Heat and stir until the wax has melted, then pour the two ingredients into a food processor. Into a small pan, pour the same amount of flower water or herbal tea as you have used of oil, adding 15 ml (1 tbsp) of the glycerine, and allow the mixture to warm through until just starting to steam.

Now back to the food processor – ensure that the oil and wax mixture is starting to turn slightly opaque but can still move freely when the food processor is on. This is the perfect stage for getting the two lots of ingredients to emulsify properly. Turn on the food processor and slowly trickle the warm tea or flower water into the oil mix, stopping periodically to scrape down the sides and ensure it mixes correctly. When all the ingredients have emulsified, add 1 ml of vitamin E per 100 ml of oil mix, and 2–3 drops of rose essential oil per 100 ml of oil mix – you can add more if you prefer, though this really depends on how strongly fragrant you want your cream to be. Give the mixture one last brief mix, then decant it into clean, dry jars. Move fairly quickly with this – the cream will set as it cools and is usually a lot more difficult to put into jars once it reaches this point!

Use this cream twice a month or more as a breast massage, perhaps at the same time as doing routine checks for any changes in breast shape or texture. This cream will tone breast tissue as well as being a wonderful part of any self-care and self-love routine. If the cream separates once it has cooled, just use a clean dry cloth or kitchen towel to wick off any extra moisture – this sometimes happens when room temperatures vary widely throughout the day, changing from cool to hot. If in doubt, store the cream in the fridge.

Lime / Linden
Tilia europaea

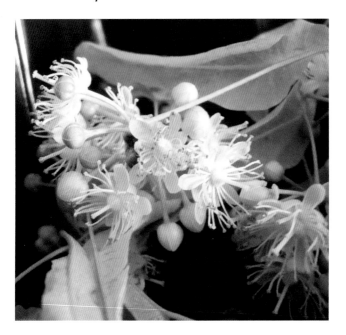

Also known as: teil, basswood

Family   Tiliaceae.

Habitat and description   The lime is a tall, stately, deciduous tree with heart-shaped, asymmetrical, elegant green leaves, the buds and young versions of which can be eaten in salads and stir fries. This long-lived tree can grow up to 40 m (130 ft) tall. The five-petalled hermaphroditic flowers are small and honey-coloured, with green bracts that help the seeds to be carried a distance away from the tree in the autumn; they form in clusters all over the branches and are much beloved by the bees that congregate around the branches during flowering season, with much busy buzzing and chattering. The flowers tend to deposit a honey sap all over the place and can cause quite a mess on cars parked underneath them! The distinctive fragrance carries quite some way in the summer and is utterly enticing, having a green, floral scent to it.

In the autumn, the seeds begin green with a velvety coating and mature into a soft golden colour before being carried away from the tree on the breeze.

Where to find it   UK and Europe, North America, Scandinavia, other temperate regions.

Parts used   Flowers gathered young, green fruits, and young leaves can be eaten.

When to gather   The young leaves can be gathered and eaten when they appear in April and early May. Gather the leaves that appear slightly translucent, as these have the best texture for eating. The flowers appear from late June to July and can be gathered as soon as they open. The very young fruit can be gathered in the early autumn.

Medicines to make   Teas and tisanes to calm the nerves; soothing baths and sleep pillows, combined with other herbs.

Constituents   Volatile oils, including geraniol and linalool; flavonoids such as quercetin; mucilage; steroidal saponins; triterpenoid saponins; phenolic and amino acids and tannins, to give a very brief outline.

Planetary influence   Venus.

Associated deities and heroes   Frigga, Laima, and probably any other Goddesses associated with birth and fertility as well as prophecy – the mother archetype, basically.

Festival   Midsummer.

Constitution   Cool and moist.

Actions and indications   Limeflower is a wonderful sedative, encouraging lower stress levels and restful sleep when drunk as a tea, or if taken as a tincture or elixir. It also has a reputation as a useful cardiovascular herb, improving circulation around the body and lowering blood pressure, particularly when high blood pressure is linked to high stress levels. It will relieve spasm and tension in the blood vessels and is also effective in relieving menopausal hypertension and anxiety.

As a cooling herb, limeflower is also superb for hot constitutions and any illness where heat trapped in the body is causing trouble. Drink the cold tea to relieve menopausal hot flushes, especially sweetened with a little limeflower honey – the honey made from limeflowers retains some of its sedative properties, making it particularly good for any stress-related issues. Why not steep limeflowers in limeflower honey to make a soothing and gently sedative syrup?

Drunk as a hot tea, it is a superb diaphoretic, helping the body to relieve and ease influenza and fevers. It can also be used to soothe irritated coughs and bronchitis, as well as to help the body get rid of excessive levels of catarrh in the

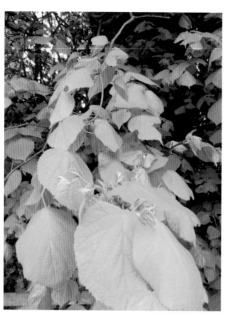

lungs, making it a lovely soothing remedy for coughs and colds, as it will help you get to sleep while also relieving the cough and calming some of the discomfort associated with the common cold or flu.

Limeflower has nervine and antispasmodic properties, making it great for the relief of stress and stress-related issues, such as anxiety and insomnia. The antispasmodic properties combine with the sedative properties to make it really helpful for the relief of headaches and migraines, especially when these are due to tension: jaw- and shoulder-tensing levels of tension that lead to headaches, in particular the sort that begin at the base of the neck and reach jagged fingers over the top of the skull, and the sort caused by jaw-clenching.

Those delicious antispasmodic properties make it handy for all sorts of spasmodic issues, including stomach cramps, chest cramps, period pains and colic.

The herb can also be used to relieve a variety of stomach issues ranging from indigestion, vomiting, IBS and diarrhoea – again especially when these are due to tension or worsened by stress levels – so consider a tea of it after a hasty lunch to help it settle correctly and calm mid-afternoon stress levels.

Externally, the tea or bath or can be used to relieve a wide variety of itchy or sore skin conditions, from bites and stings to sores and abscesses. Make basins of infusion from the flowers to add to a warm bath to relieve stress and anxiety. I suspect the flower water could also be used for this, and the essential oil is certainly relaxing and calming.

Folklore   The inner bark can be used to make a variety of items, including clothes, shoes, ropes, mats and nets.

According to folklore, one ancient linden tree planted in the year 1000 finally died in the 1900s, and there are copses of linden trees in Europe that are hundreds, if not over a thousand years old.

The wood is lightweight and dense but flexible and has long been used to make shields, and for carving statues and figurines. The tree is by its very nature strongly linked to both joy and protection – a strong yet maternal presence in our hedgerows, gardens and woods. Standing under a linden tree in full bloom is an utterly intoxicating experience that I highly recommend.

Dose   Ten ml (2 tsp) of the tincture or elixir taken up to twice a day, or 5 ml (1 tsp), heaped, of the chopped dried herb to a cup of hot water, steeped for 5 minutes and drunk up to three times a day.

Steep large quantities of the dried or fresh flowers in jugs of just-boiled water and add them to a bath – but remember to filter out the flowers first or risk blocking the plug!

Contraindications   Older flowers are narcotic and should not be gathered from the tree. Pick them young instead.

Limeflower recipes

Limeflower herbal honey

This honey is really very simple to make, and if you can possibly manage it, source some limeflower honey for the recipe – local farmers markets may have it, as may the local farm shops and health food shops. Simply gather young flowers from the tree, avoiding the bees who will certainly give you annoyed looks as you do, and roughly chop them, or even use them whole. Pile the flowers into a clean jar and pour over enough honey to cover them, with a little extra honey on top. Stir the whole lot gently to ensure the honey has covered all the plant matter, then put the lid on and leave it to infuse.

Add this honey to calming teas, have 5 ml (1 tsp) to calm mid-afternoon ab-dabs, or use it over puddings, sponges and pancakes as a delicious and calming sweet treat. You could even use it on the skin, if needed – smear some over a large, clean plaster and apply it over abscesses and boils to help them drain and heal.

Limeflower aromatic water

Preparing this aromatic water is rather more complex, requiring the use of an alembic, if you can get one. These are now available in all sorts of sizes, ranging from a ½-litre pot all the way up to a huge 5-gallon affair: larger ones are required for creating essential oils, while the smaller ones work beautifully for making aromatic waters at home.

Ingredients / equipment
  » at least 1 pint of limeflowers, picked fresh if possible
  » enough water to cover the flowers
  » plenty of water to keep the receiving pot cool
  » a source of heat – a camping stove works well!
  » rye (or any other grain) flour and water to make a thick paste used to seal the alembic
  » a small alembic – 1.5 litres for the main pot is plenty large enough for home use, unless you have a lot of aromatic plants and you want to have a go at making essential oils as well
  » one large jug and one small jug
  » a decent long length of pipe with a tap on the end – have a look in home brewing and cooking shops, as the sets of pipe, tap and rigid tube for racking-off wine work beautifully for this. I cut a 25-cm (10-in.) piece off one end to put on the front of the receiving vessel and use the rest for swapping out the water in the pot itself

Instructions   Alembics are surprisingly easy to use, for all that they look rather imposing when you first catch sight of them! They usually separate into three pieces: an onion-shaped base pot, the cap and a long stem, and the receiving vessel. Gather the limeflowers and pack them into the main pot, then cover them with enough water to just obscure the flowers before putting the top on with its pipe.

Mix up rye flour with just enough water to make a really thick doughy paste, and pack a thick layer of this around the join between the bottom of the pot and the top with its long spout on, then connect the end of this pipe to the top of the receiving vessel, repeating the process with the dough mix to seal the join. You do this to stop any steam from escaping, as the steam contains the aromatic oils that you want to hang on to.

Put the large pot onto the camping stove or on top of the cooker, and turn on the heat, making sure that the receiving pot is at the same level as the stove, so that the whole apparatus sits on the same level. Make sure the receiving vessel is filled with cold water – ice cubes work well, as they will hang on to the cool temperature for that little bit longer. Ideally you will have a tap adaptor and pipe to connect the tap to the top of the alembic: this makes the whole job a lot easier, as you can have one pipe bringing cool water into the top of the receiving vessel and another pipe removing warm water from the bottom of it into the sink or a demijohn underneath. I use a large jug or a large bottle of water and keep a steady trickle running into the receiving vessel that way, though this does make for a lot more work. Setting up next to the kitchen sink is ideal if you have the space!

You will find that it will take a few minutes for the pot to start to boil, and you can feel the copper start to warm up as the steam moves along it – be careful with how and when you touch the copper pot, as it will get very hot, copper being a really good conductor of heat! Make sure you have a small pipe connected to the bottom of the receiving vessel that runs into a jug for the aromatic water to run into. I use the pipe from a set for racking-off home brew and find this works admirably! Once the water starts to boil, turn the heat under the pot right down. If the pot boils too quickly and too furiously, it can force the herb tea up the tube and right over into the receiving pot, which rather spoils the resulting herb water.

Keep the cool water trickling into the receiving vessel so that the pipes remain cold, and then it is simply a waiting game, keeping an eye on the receiving jug with the aromatic water in it. I suggest measuring how much water you put into the main pot before you turn the heat on, so that you can keep track of how much aromatic water you can expect to get out of the end!

The resulting aromatic water can be used as a toner on the skin, as a spray on bites and stings, or as an ingredient in healing creams and lotions; it should keep for up to a year in a cool cupboard, though it smells so good I suspect you will use it up long before then.

Limeflower and honeysuckle elixir

Ingredients
- » plenty of limeflowers
- » one bottle of vodka
- » local honey

Instructions   Another very simple recipe to make – just pile the flowers into a clean Kilner jar, pour over plenty of vodka, and add 2–3 tbsp of local honey. If you can get limeflower honey, so much the better, but any good honey will work well for this recipe. Let the whole lot steep for at least two weeks – you can continue to add fresh flowers throughout this time if you want to, though I would recommend leaving it for at least another week once the last lot of flowers has gone in. Strain out the herbs and enjoy 10 ml (2 tsp) in a pretty glass when feeling stressed out or suffering with a tension headache, or if struggling with the midsummer heat. This will also help to relieve the symptoms of coughs and colds, again being well suited to the summer cold. I have recommended vodka over brandy for this recipe as this has a mild-enough flavour to really allow the gorgeously aromatic scented herbs to fully express themselves in the finished elixir.

Why not try using this as part of a mixer cocktail, adding elderflower cordial and either sugar-free lemonade or fizzy water?

Limeflower tea

There are two versions of this recipe: if using the resulting tea as a wash or bath, simply pile plenty of fresh herbs into a bowl or cafetiere, and pour over enough hot water to cover them amply. Put a lid on the bowl – if you let too much steam escape, those gorgeous volatile oils will fly away with it. Let the whole lot steep until cool, then strain out the flowers and add to the bath, or use as a skin wash.

For a version that you can drink, put 1 tsp of roughly chopped flowers into a cup, pour over enough hot water to fill the vessel, and then put a saucer over the whole thing – remember those volatile oils! Let the tea infuse for 5–10 minutes before drinking. If you are trying to break a fever, drink as hot as you can stand, otherwise you can let it cool down completely if you want to, before drinking it.

Meadowsweet
Filipendula ulmaria

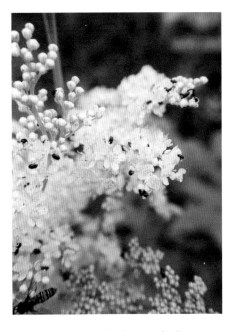

Also known as: queen of the meadow, bridewort, little queen, gravel root, trumpet weed, lady of the meadow, steeplebush, bride of the meadow, meadsweet, mead wort, pride of the meadow, meadow maid, honeysweet, dollor, meadow wort, bridgewort, dollof, lace-makers-herb

Family Rosaceae.

Habitat and description Meadowsweet (*Filipendula ulmaria*, previously known as *Spiraea ulmaria*) likes to grow with its feet wet and can often be found on wetland, by rivers, and on commons and boggy ground. It also grows in or near ditches alongside fields and is a familiar sight in the countryside,

95

where it is clearly visible in the flowering season as it edges fields, ditches and hedgerows. We have a plethora of it growing in and around our village, with more and more appearing each year, so we won't run out for a while yet!

The leaves are roughly diamond-shaped, deeply grooved and toothed around the edges, with a fairly rigid set to them, growing in pairs up a slender stem, with one leaf at the apex. The central stem is often reddish in colour, and the whole plant, which tends to be low-growing until flowering, can grow up to about 50 cm to 1 m (2–4 ft) tall. The flowers are creamy-coloured and have a slightly feathery appearance. They are strongly fragrant and have been used in brewing and cooking since time immemorial. The whole plant in flower is a beautiful sight, well deserving of the title 'Queen of the Meadow'. The leaves have a distinctive, medicinal scent to them when bruised and make a pleasant-tasting tea.

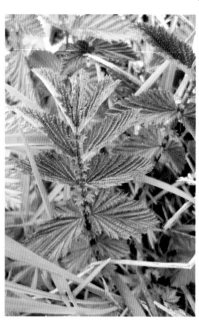

Where to find it   UK and Europe, parts of Asia and the East, North America.

Parts used   The whole herb, used in flower, and the flowers used separately to make oils.

When to gather   I have gathered the leaves year round and made useful medicines from them, but I find the ones gathered while the plant is in flower to be the most effective for acid digestion and related issues. The flowers are gathered from July to early September. In April and May, the young leaves make a delicious tea.

Medicines to make   Infused oils, balms and salves with the flowers, for sore muscles, aches and strains; teas, tinctures and elixirs with the whole plant, for digestive issues and suchlike.

Constituents   The plant contains a variety of constituents, including volatile oils (including up to 75% salicylaldehyde); phenolic glycosides, including spiraein and gaultherin; flavonoids; tannins (predominantly hydrolysable); traces of coumarin and ascorbic acid.

Planetary influence   Jupiter (although, typically enough, our old friend Culpeper disagrees and states that it is ruled by Venus. Since these two planets are fairly similar in terms of both being fairly mild and expansive, I don't think it really makes much difference.)

Associated deities and heroes   Blodeuwedd, Aine, Gwena, Venus. Other women who could be considered to be Flowerbrides, such as Guinevere; considering the long association of meadowsweet with Faerie, its possible other faery deities could be listed here such as Morgana, Mab and Titania, and, of course, other Goddesses associated with love and beauty – such as Freyja and Aphrodite.

Festival   Midsummer.

Constitution   Cool and dry.

Actions and indications   Culpeper used to use the herb to dry the body out and to stop bleeding, diarrhoea, vomiting and excessive menstruation. He also reckoned that it can be used to 'make a merry heart' and comments that the leaf or flower can be added to claret wine for this purpose. If this mix is drunk warm with some honey added, it can relieve constipation, but drunk cold, it stops diarrhoea. Externally he states that it can be used to treat sores, cankers and fistulas, and the distilled water can be used to treat heat and inflammatory conditions in the eyes (one can assume he possibly means conjunctivitis). I would suggest making an aromatic water of the herb using an alembic as well, for topical use – for instructions on this, please refer to the section on limeflower.

Gerard really didn't use the herb much, although he does clarify Culpeper's comment regarding the eyes, mentioning that the flower water relieves burning and itching and clears the sight. He mentions that meadowsweet is an excellent strewing herb, and that the scent of the flower gladdens the heart.

Most folks tend to focus on the herb's use for gastrointestinal problems, including gastric and peptic ulceration, acid reflux, diarrhoea, liver disorders and related problems, as well as urinary disorders such as cystitis, and reddish deposits in the urine with an accompanying oily film, and urinary stones. I certainly have the most experience using this herb internally for acid digestion, indigestion, hangover, peptic ulceration and any other hot, overly acidic condition of the digestive tract, for which it can often feel like a miracle cure. It is amphoteric, meaning that it balances acid production. If the body is producing too much, it eases back the amount. If it is producing too little, meadowsweet encourages the body to produce a bit more.

As the whole plant contains salicylic acid (one of the original precursors of aspirin) it can also be used as a mild to moderate painkiller, relieving all sorts of musculoskeletal aches and discomforts as well as the muscle aches linked with influenza and the common cold, mild neuralgias and joint-aches. It has been used in the past to treat gout, though given that a lot of the time salicylic acid doesn't suit gouty consti-tutions well, use it with caution if you plan to give this a try.

The whole plant is an aromatic stomach tonic, anti-inflam-matory, astringent and antibacterial – a handy addition to the medicine cupboard!

The plant does have some immunostimulant action through the herb's liver tonic and digestive stimulant action, and the whole plant is a strong diuretic and urinary antiseptic, as well as being a useful painkiller that can treat headaches and assorted pains associated with the joint system. The flowers can be used fresh or dried as a diaphoretic, and apparently the plant has been used successfully in some cases concern-ing weight gain where this has been caused by problems with fat metabolism.

I tend to gather and use the whole plant in flower, both infusing the flowers in oil to make a muscle rub for sore muscles, neck ache and rheumatism, and drying the flowers and leaves to use as a tea. It also makes a beautiful spagyric tincture, with a deep, rich red colour.

Folklore   Meadowsweet is one of the three herbs held to be sacred by the Druids, the other two being vervain and water mint. In more recent history, the plant used to be known as *Spiraea ulmaria* and is the plant from which the original aspirin was derived, as it has high levels of salicylic acid, an anodyne.

The plant was historically used to flavour mead, hence the folk name of 'mead wort'. It was a popular strewing flower and was often used in bridal bouquets and posies.

Apparently it was given to Cuchulainn to calm his fits of rage and outbreaks of fever, as is shown in the plant's Gaelic name, 'belt of Cuchulainn'. This is interesting as the plant is cool and dry and could certainly be useful in the easing of more choleric problems, such as anger! Anger in and of itself isn't a big problem, but the negative expression of it can cause huge issues for some people.

The plant has a strong association with death, and in folklore the scent of the flowers could induce a deep and fatal sleep under some circumstances. Some say that the plant was given its scent by the Moon Goddess Aine. Apparently the flowers used to be dried and smoked in Nottinghamshire, where they gained the name 'Old Man's Pepper', after the Devil: interesting, given that it was probably less damaging to the health than tobacco is!

Dose   I tend to use up to 5 ml (1 tsp) three times a day if needed but prefer giving this herb as a tea for digestive issues; 1 tsp of dried herb to a cup of hot water, steeped for 5 minutes and drunk up to three times a day, should suffice.

Contraindications   Those allergic to aspirin shouldn't risk taking this herb. Use it with some care if you have gout – this ailment doesn't often play well with salicylic acid.

Meadowsweet recipes

Peppermint and meadowsweet pills for stomach aches and acid indigestion

Ingredients
 » dried peppermint – at least 20 g
 » dried meadowsweet – at least 20 g
 » local runny honey
 » arrowroot powder

Instructions   Powder the peppermint and meadowsweet as much as you possibly can using a herb grinder followed by a mortar and pestle – the finer the powder, the more pleasant the final stomach pills will be to take. Put the powdered herbs into a large bowl and add 1 tbsp of arrowroot powder, stir this in thoroughly and add 5 ml (1 tsp) of local runny honey and, using the teaspoon, mash and work the herbs into the honey. Add more honey if you find that you have plenty of herbs left over, in ⅓-of-a-teaspoon increments. Keep working the herbs and honey mixture together until you have a thick paste: add more arrowroot if you need to get a thicker consistency. If need be, you can transfer the whole lot into a smooth-sided mortar and use the pestle to work the ingredients together.

Next, spread out some greaseproof paper onto a baking tray and, using your fingertips, form the mixture into tiny balls about the size of a pea, rolling them in more arrowroot at the end if you need to. Drop them onto the baking sheet, making sure that they do not touch each other. Once the sheet is full, preheat the oven to around 80°C and pop the tray in. Check your pills every half hour – they tend to take approximately 2 hours to bake at this temperature. You can also use a dehydrator on the highest setting for this purpose. Once the pills have cooled, they should set hard and be crunchy. Store them in an airtight container and take up to 4 pills to relieve nausea, upset stomach, wind and bloating. Crunch them up, or swallow them whole, with some water, if preferred.

Meadowsweet, honeysuckle and feverfew headache elixir or honegar

Ingredients
- » 1 pint, loosely packed, each, of meadowsweet flowering tops, honeysuckle flowers and feverfew leaves
- » vodka or brandy or unpasteurised cider vinegar
- » local honey

Instructions As usual, check over your plant parts for bird poop and any unhealthy-looking bits, then finely chop them. Pack them into a Kilner jar and pour over enough vodka or brandy or cider vinegar to cover the plant matter with about 2.5 cm (1 in.) on top, then dollop in at least 1 heaped table-spoonful of local honey, stirring it in thoroughly. Put the lid on and shake the mixture up, then pack the plant matter back down under the level of the alcohol. Pop the lid on and let it steep for a fortnight, then strain out the herbs. A good dosage for this is 5 ml (1 tsp) as needed, up to three times a day. This is particularly good for heat-related headaches. If your headaches are more stress-related, consider including some German chamomile flowers as well, so use ⅔ of a pint of each plant instead of a full pint of three of them.

Meadowsweet-flower infused oil

Ingredients / equipment
- » 1 pint of meadowsweet flower heads, gently pressed down in the jug
- » 500 ml (17½ fl oz) sunflower seed oil
- » double boiler

Instructions De–bug the flower heads – a task best done outdoors, especially on a stormy day, as there will be quite a lot of thunderflies sitting among the creamy flowers. If you can, put them in a basket in a shady place – most of the time the small passengers will vacate the flowers and head out the nearest window or door. Put the flowers in the top of the double boiler and cover with the oil, then put the double boiler on a medium heat until the water has come to a gentle simmer. Turn the heat down and allow to bubble quietly for up to an hour, then turn off and leave to cool. Strain out the flowers and the murky oil at the bottom, and bottle the rest. This can be applied to sore joints and muscles, as well as trapped nerves, and is a wonderful painkiller and anti-inflammatory. Meadowsweet flowers are generally ready for picking between July and August and can be found growing in many hedgerows around Lincolnshire.

Meadowsweet spagyric tincture – a brief introduction

Ingredients / equipment
- » two large bunches of meadowsweet gathered when in flower and dried down
- » vodka or brandy
- » a heat source – camping stove, outdoor fire pit or anything like that will work well

Instructions This is a complicated but rather fascinating medicine to make. Try to gather the meadowsweet at the appropriate time of day and week (this is a very complicated subject in itself, and as a rough guide I suggest gathering it on a Wednesday where possible, in the middle of the day when the energy of the plant is at its highest. You can get even more complicated than this by figuring out where the planets are and picking accordingly, but this is far beyond the remit of this book.)

Dry one of the bunches of meadowsweet thoroughly, a process that will take between a week and a month depending on the time of year and where it is hanging. With the other, make up a tincture by finely chopping the herbs, piling them into a Kilner jar, and pouring over plenty of the alcohol. Two to three weeks later, the herbs can be strained out of the alcohol and pressed thoroughly. Don't throw this "marque" away – you will need it later! Thoroughly chop or shred the dried meadowsweet and pack both this and the spent marque from the tincture into a large saucepan or pot that can withstand plenty of intense heat. This where it gets fun – now the whole pot needs to be put on a heat source – outdoors, as this part of the process generates a lot of smoke. Burn the herbs thoroughly until they go black and stop smoking, then continue to burn them until they turn white. You should be left with a small amount of white ash, which should be given time to totally cool. To this add 2 litres of distilled water or collected dew, and simmer gently for around 20–30 minutes; cool, then strain the whole lot into a large bowl through a muslin cloth or filter paper. What is left of the ash in the filter paper or cloth is the caput mortuum, or death's head, which can be disposed of. The remaining water needs to be simmered down gently at a point just below boiling until white crystals are left in the bottom of the pan. Repeat the process again with another equal amount of water, straining it again to make sure the crystals are as pure as possible. Once you are left with fine white crystals in the bottom of the pan – and they are small, I warn you now – I recommend pouring the tincture straight over the crystals once the pan is cool, mix it up thoroughly, and then bottle it, leaving it in a warm, dark place for a fortnight.

The final step is to put the tincture somewhere that will get warm during the day and return it to a fridge at night – this activates the resulting liquid, rendering it more potent. This tincture can be used in much smaller doses than the standard ones and is a truly magical thing in its own right – begin at 1 drop in a little water, and work up to 7 drops with time. This is, by necessity, a brief introduction to spagyric tincture making – check the bibliography at the back for more in-depth books on the subject.

Mugwort
Artemisia vulgaris

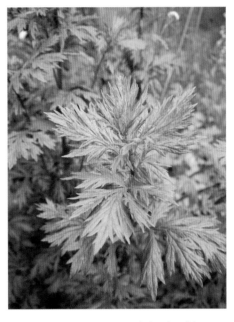

Also known as: artemisia, witch herb, old man,
old uncle harry, artemis herb, muggons, sailor's tobacco, apple
pie, mugger, smotherwort, felon herb, St Johns plant, cingulum
sancti, johannis, mother's wort, maiden wort, muggins

Family   Asteraceae.

Habitat and description   Mugwort is a perennial that grows
to approximately 1.2 m (4 ft) tall, with a downy, slightly silvery
appearance to the leaves. The leaves are deeply pinnate, with
up to seven lobes that are deeply cut and dark green on the
top, with few hairs. The undersides are silvery, and the whole

plant is aromatic to the touch, especially in late summer during flowering, when the scent is at its most intense.

The flowers are yellowish green in colour, small and fairly insignificant, and blossom in tall, branched spikes. The plant is found throughout Europe and is even considered a weed in some places, as it does tend to rather take over when it gets a foothold and self-seeds readily. The plant tends to prefer disturbed soil and waste ground to grow on, but will do well in normal garden soil. I have found a lot of it near the river, and it would seem that the plant is quite amenable to growing with its feet wet if necessary, though it is usually to be found by waysides and hedgerows, waving its silver undersides at people with wild abandon on windy days.

Where to find it   UK and Europe; North America; Asia; parts of Africa.

Parts used   Aerial parts.

When to gather   July and August when it is in flower, which is usually when it is at its most aromatic.

Medicines to make   Digestive and mood-boosting elixirs and

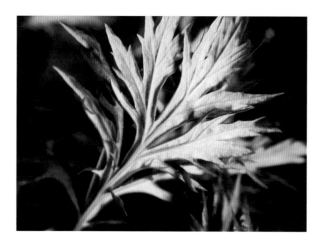

tinctures, infused oils, sleep pillows, dried herb as a tea or incense, smudge sticks.

Constituents   A range of volatile oils, such as alpha and beta thujone and other oils, sesquiterpene lactones, including vulgarin, pilostachyn and others; flavonoids, coumarin derivatives, including umbelliferone, aesculentin, and also caffeic acid derivatives, as well as some triterpenes.

Planetary influence   The Moon / Venus.

Star sign   Taurus / Libra.

Associated deities   Pretty much all of the Moon Goddesses, as well as quite a few of the deities linked with witchcraft.

Festival   Midsummer is the traditional association, but I also link it with Samhain, due to its long link with prophecy and divination.

Constitution   Warm and dry.

Actions and indications   Mugwort has a wide range of medicinal uses, only a tiny few of which we seem to take advantage of these days. It has a range of antibacterial and antifungal properties, making it handy for skin washes and balms as well as internally to help the body heal from infection or fungal overgrowth, such as candida or thrush. It contains a wide variety of aromatic oils, giving it some useful digestive properties as a stomach tonic and gall-bladder and pancreas tonic. It has been used in the past as a mild sedative, as well as to boost and lift the mood gently – I tend to use it to stabilise those who are prone to mood swings, whether this is due to digestive issues or to just how they are emotionally.

It is a gentle nervous system stimulant and has been used to relieve digestive tension and improve digestive regulation – quite probably due to the bitter taste, which stimulates the vagus nerve, which, in turn, benefits the digestive system. It has been linked with female sex hormones and to excessive androgen production, making it a useful herb for polycystic ovary syndrome (PCOS) and related issues. A standard indication for mugwort is a weaker pulse in the right wrist than there is in the left, indicating that the masculine impulses have overwhelmed the feminine principles. Mugwort could be considered an excellent herb to bring about balance.

It has been used previously as an anti-diabetic, perhaps due to its stomachic properties, as well as a gentle diuretic, and to bring on delayed periods and for extreme period pain, though it should be used with caution if pregnancy is suspected and should be avoided if pregnancy has been confirmed.

It is a wonderful herb for relieving nervous tension; it has also been used for the symptomatic relief of Parkinson's tremor as well as for epilepsy and convulsions. As a tea, it can relieve insomnia as well as shaking anxiety, making it a delicious way to calm down from mid-afternoon stress.

It has been used in the past as a strong blood cleanser, which some even consider to be on a par with herbs such as *echinacea*. I combine it with elderberry and nettle for this purpose.

It is a gentle diuretic as well as being a blood cleanser and antibacterial, so a tea of it can be used to help the body to recover from cystitis or any infection of the womb.

A tincture of mugwort can be used to encourage more vivid dreams for some people, while in others already struggling with disturbed sleep due to dreaming, it can downgrade the dreams and allow a better quality of rest.

Folklore   The herb was known as *Cingulum Sancti Johannis*, or 'St John's Girdle', in the Middle Ages, as legend has it that St John the Baptist wore a girdle of mugwort while he was in the wilderness. It was also traditionally worn on Midsummer's Eve as a garland while dancing around the fire. Afterwards it was thrown onto the fire to protect the wearer from danger and sickness throughout the year. Interestingly, mugwort has been used, much as elder has, both to protect the wearer from witchcraft and also as an ingredient in the magic of witches. The juice of the plant was used to anoint scrying devices to aid in divination. Another old piece of Germanic folklore reckons that a rare coal can be found under mugwort, but only during one hour of one specific day of the year – some versions of the legend state that this is noon on Midsummer's Day. If this coal is put under the pillow, it will bring about dreams of a future husband. The coal in question is a certain remedy against evil and may even become gold. In ancient days the herb was known as 'Mater Herbarum' (the mother of herbs).

The Anglo-Saxons knew of mugwort and revered it – it is one of the nine sacred herbs mentioned in the *Lacnunga*, an ancient text on Anglo-Saxon herbalism. 'Eldest of worts, thou hast might for three, and against thirty, for venom availest, for flying vile things, might against loathed ones that through the land rove.' Perhaps an early reference to airborne bacteria.

There is an old Russian folktale about mugwort, known in Russian as *Zabytko*. Apparently a young girl, gathering mushrooms in the forest, fell into a deep pit, which turned out to be the home of snakes. The snakes did not harm her and took care of her throughout the winter, during which time both she and the snakes got their nourishment from a mysterious glowing stone (a possible allusion to the moon)? When spring finally arrived, the snakes formed a ladder with their bodies, allowing the girl to climb out, and, as a parting gift, the Serpent Queen taught her the language of the plants, but warned that if she should ever call mugwort by name, she would immediately lose the ability. A long time afterwards, she was walking with her lover along a footpath when he asked her the name of a tall herb growing by the wayside. Without thinking, she answered 'mugwort' and immediately forgot the language of plants. The Russians know mugwort as the herb of forgetfulness.

Dose   I tend to use 1 tsp, lightly heaped, of the dried herb to a cup of hot water, steeped and drunk up to three times a day. For the tincture, no more than 5 ml (1 tsp) up to twice a day.

Contraindications   Do not take mugwort during pregnancy. The herb can cause contact dermatitis in some people, especially those with an allergy to the daisy family.

Mugwort recipes

Mugwort and sage smudge sticks

Ingredients / equipment
- » fresh mugwort leaves gathered on a dry day – smaller stems are fine as well
- » fresh sage – purple or white works fine, whichever you have in the garden
- » cotton yarn or string for binding

Instructions   To make sure the surface of your herbs is completely dry, pick on a dry, sunny day after the dew has evaporated off. Make a small, narrow pile of the mugwort on a clean, dry surface, layering in sage leaves alternately with the mugwort leaves; then, using some cotton string or yarn, tie a tight loop around one end of the bundle, keeping a firm grip on it and leaving a good 5 cm (2 in.) free so that you can tie off the yarn at the end.

Wind the yarn up the length of the stick tightly, making sure at least five loops encircle the stick from one end to the other, then wrap it around at least half a dozen times, pulling it tightly each time, to form a good layer of yarn at the other end. Once you have done this, wind it around back up the length of the stick, until you reach your starting point again, giving it another half-dozen tight loops close together at this end. Tie it off tightly. Put the smudge stick in a cool, dry place with good ventilation, and make sure you turn it over regularly, so that it dries evenly. Light one end of the stick and allow it to smoulder as you cleanse the energies of a place.

Mugwort bitters

Ingredients
  » plenty of fresh mugwort leaves gathered while the plant is in flower
  » orange, lemon or lime zest
  » cider vinegar

Instructions   Thoroughly chop the herbs and the zest and pile them into a Kilner jar, pouring over plenty of vinegar. Seal and leave the whole lot to infuse for at least a fortnight, then strain out the herbs. Add 5 ml (1 tsp) of the bitters to a small glass of water, to be sipped before meals. This will encourage better digestion and appetite.

Mugwort and hop sleep pillows

Ingredients / equipment
  » plenty of well-dried mugwort in flower, thoroughly chopped up
  » dried hops – an equal amount to the mugwort
  » cotton – not too fine, as you don't want stray mugwort stems poking you in the face while you try to sleep!
  » needle and thread
  » lavender essential oil if preferred

Instructions   Cut a rectangle of the fabric, in a size that suits you, then fold it in half and sew around two of the open sides to create an open pouch. Turn the pouch inside out, stuff it thoroughly with the chopped, mixed herbs and essential oils, then carefully turn the open top edge inwards and sew it closed. This can be put in the pillow, or under the pillow, and will encourage sleep and for some people, more vivid dreams.

Mugwort tea

This tea is very easy to make, and can use either fresh or dried herbs. Simply allow 1 tsp, heaped, of fresh herbs or one slightly domed teaspoon of dried herbs to a cup of hot water, cover and infuse for 5 minutes. Drink when feeling stressed out or wound up, and to settle an over-full or uncomfortable stomach.

Mullein
Verbascum thapsus

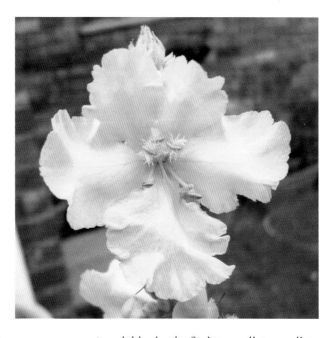

Also known as: aaron's rod, blanket leaf, white mullein, mullein
dock, Our Lady's flannel, blanket herb, woollen, rag paper, wild
ice leaf, clown's lungwort, bullock's lungwort, beggar's staff,
goldenrod, adam's flannel, beggar's blanket, cuddy's lungs,
fluffweed, feltwort, hare's beard, candlewick plant, clot, doffle,
feltwort, flannel plant, graveyard dust, hag's tapers, hedge taper,
jupiter's staff, lady's foxglove, old man's flannel, peter's staff,
shepherd's club, shepherd's herb, torches, velvetback, velvet plant

Family   Scrophulariaceae.

Habitat and description   As you can no doubt guess by the
wide variety of colourful and descriptive nicknames for this

tall, stately plant, mullein has decidedly hairy leaves, covered
in a soft, silvery-coloured down. The leaves themselves grow
in rosettes around the stem and are large and oval in shape,
a soft pale green-grey in colour. The flowers grow on a tall
stem rising many feet above the leaves, with randomly placed,
honey-fragranced yellow flowers growing in profusion up the
stem – these appear in the second year of growth. It prefers
a well-drained soil that tends towards dryness and can be a
bit tricky to grow in the herb garden as a result – I find it
a bit hit and miss at times for this exact reason. The flower
spikes sometimes divide at the top into smaller flower-laden
branches. The plant itself is a biennial. It can be found on
sunny banks, fields, roadsides and in wasteland, preferring a
poor, dry, chalky soil for best growth. It grows in profusion
in Suffolk, where I spent most of my childhood.

Where to find it   Europe, North Africa, and parts of Asia;
it has also been introduced into parts of Australia and the
Americas.

Parts used   Aerial parts – leaves and flowers. The roots are
also sometimes used.

When to gather   The leaves are gathered in the first year
for teas and tinctures to ease mucous membrane issues; the

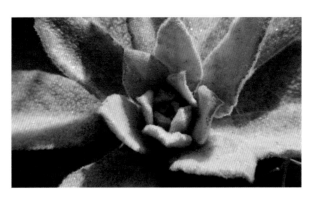

flowers are gathered in the second year and used to make infused oils for ear problems. If you are using the roots, gather them in the autumn or winter after the first year of growth.

Medicines to make   Infused oil of the flowers for ear problems and nerve issues; teas and tinctures for lung and stomach issues; infused oils and balms for use as poultices.

Constituents   Iridoids, including ajugol; flavonoids such as verbascoside; saponins; volatile oils; tannins; mucilage.

Planetary influence   Saturn.

Associated deities and heroes   Jupiter, Circe, Odysseus, St. Fiacre. Given the folklore and alternative names for this plant, I suspect one could probably associate it with assorted crone deities and death deities as well.

Festival   Samhain.

Constitution   Cool and moist, but only slightly so: generally temperate.

Actions and indications   Being a classic herb of Saturn, mullein is used to restore balance and bring structure back to the body. It is used for conditions where the body has either worn down villi and tissues, resulting in harsh, dried-out conditions, or, for the other side of the coin, for problems causing the body to be saturated with too much fluid, such as oedema and mucus building up in the digestive tract and respiratory system.

The root is used by herbalists in North America to soothe acute pain. The flowers are particularly good for earache and problems affecting the nerves, whereas the leaves are better for the respiratory system and related disorders and for musculoskeletal issues.

As a softening, soothing herb, it is wonderful for longlasting, dry, tickly coughs and conditions of the lungs where the lining has worn down, resulting in regular chest infections with a tight chest, dry membranes and a chronic cough.

Mullein softens the membranes, opens the chest and allows proper breathing, acting as a tonic to the respiratory tract and alleviating the misery of winter chest infections.

The other area that mullein particularly suits is conditions affecting the joints – hot, dry, constricted conditions, such as rheumatism, arthritis and related joint complaints, as well as broken bones, strained tendons and ligaments and torn muscles – I rather suspect it will combine particularly well with comfrey for this. Indeed, it has such a long-standing reputation in this area that even Culpeper recommended it as useful for gout and stiff sinews, as well as for dislocated joints and broken bones.

Mullein can also be used as a painkiller and nervine, soothing and easing conditions where the nerves have become trapped and tight. The flowers can be used as a mild sedative for insomnia – another usage linking the flowers to the nerves: quite appropriate, really, when you consider the structure of the plant and where the flowers are located – right at the very top of the stem.

Mullein can also be used to ease both acute and chronic cystitis and to relieve water retention and bladder irritation. As a useful digestive remedy, it can be used for those suffering from abdominal pain, diarrhoea with urgency and long-lasting digestive upset.

The flowers infused in seed oil is a useful remedy for earache and ear infections when rubbed around the base of the ear and 1–2 drops placed into the ear itself – not recommended, however, if you have a perforated ear drum.

Topically, mullein can be used to make a great drawing poultice or ointment for splinters and bites and can be used to soothe rashes, cuts and grazes and, of course, to ease the pain from broken bones and dislocated joints.

Folklore   Some think that the Latin name *Verbascum* is a corruption of the original word for beard, *barba*, alluding to the woolly appearance of the plant. The plant was certainly known by the Greeks and Romans – Pliny suggested that figs should be wrapped in mullein leaves to help them keep fresh for longer. The stems were used as replacement torches by legionaries and were dipped in wax and used as candles at funerals – this usage continued up until the Middle Ages. The flowers were used by Roman women to make a blonde hairwash.

Apparently both Circe and Odysseus used the plant – Circe as part of her spells, and Odysseus to protect himself from her spells, amusingly enough!

In the Middle Ages, mullein was grown in monastery gardens as a protection from the devil. Again, conversely, mullein was used as candles in witches' spells, though if the plant was gathered in a particular set of circumstances – the sun in Virgo and the moon in Aries – the plant could be used to guard the bearer against sorcery.

The leaf has been used for hygiene purposes as well, as nappies or nappy liners, and also as toilet paper.

Dose   Up to 5 ml (1 tsp) three times a day of the tincture, or one cup of hot water over 2 tsp of the dried leaf or flower, infused for up to 15 minutes and drunk three times a day.

Contraindications   If using any of the plant as a tea, strain the resulting liquid through muslin, as the hairs growing on the leaves irritate the mouth.

Mullein recipes

Mullein flower infused oil for ear issues

Ingredients
- » plenty of mullein flowers, preferably freshly gathered
- » organic seed oil

Instructions   This can be made either on the hob, or in a jar on the windowsill and infused by the sun. If using the hob, make sure the flowers are dry, pile them into a double boiler, cover with oil, and simmer gently for at least an hour, until the oil turns bright yellow. If using a jam jar on a windowsill, pile the surface-dry flowers into the jar, cover with the oil, and fasten a piece of kitchen roll over the top to allow water to evaporate. Leave it on a hot, sunny windowsill until the oil colour has changed. This oil can be used around and in the ear itself to relieve ear pain, though avoid if you have a perforated ear drum – just massage it around the outside in this case. As a nervine, this could very probably also be combined with St John's wort as a balm for nerve pain and sciatica.

Mullein leaf tincture

Ingredients
  » plenty of fresh mullein leaves, or dried if you can't get hold of fresh ones
  » vodka or brandy – as strong as you can get hold of

Instructions   Thoroughly chop the fresh leaves and pile them into a Kilner jar. Pour over plenty of alcohol, allowing about an extra 2.5 cm (1 in.) on top, then put the lid on. Leave it in a cool, dark place to infuse for at least a fortnight, shaking it up every other day, then filter out the herbs, and bottle the remaining tincture. A good dosage would be up to 10 ml (2 tsp) three times a day for lung and digestive issues, to soothe mucous membranes – start off with a lower dose of 5 ml (1 tsp), and build up to a bigger one if the smaller quantity doesn't do the job.

Mullein root tincture

This tincture is effectively very similar to the above recipe – dig up the roots of the plant at the end of its first year, scrub them thoroughly, chop them and pile them into the brandy or vodka, leaving them to infuse for at least a fortnight. Strain out the roots and bottle. Start off with 1 ml for pain, up to three times a day, working up from there.

Pellitory-of-the-wall
Parietaria diffusa

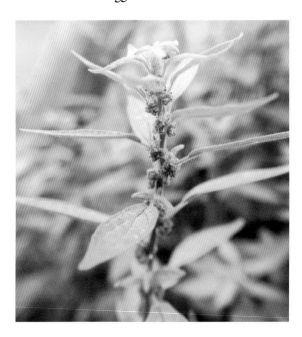

Also known as: lichwort

Family Urticaceae.

Habitat and description This often unobtrusive plant loves to grow in old walls, in cracks between the pavement and in the middle of piles of stone and rubble, sprawling in profusion. I have found it growing in numerous old abbeys and castles around the UK, where it creeps between the stones and clings with gravity-defying aplomb metres above any onlookers. A member of the nettle family, it doesn't much resemble its cousin, the stinging nettle, but instead has an upright reddish stem and gently ovate leaves that are 2½–5 cm (1–2 in.) in length in larger plants, but can be much smaller than that. The tops of the leaves are smooth but the underside is often gently furry along the veins, as is the stem. The flowers are fairly insignificant until you look closely, as so many herbal flowers are, but are surprisingly beautiful close up.

Where to find it   There are quite a few members of this particular group of plants, and they can be found over most of the world, including Europe, the Mediterranean, parts of the USA and even tropical climates.

Parts used   Aerial parts.

When to gather   When in flower.

Medicines to make   Tinctures and dried herb for tea to ease bladder and kidney issues; infused oils and balms; decoctions; poultices. Fresh juice or tea from the fresh plant is considered the best method of preparation, and I suggest tincturing fresh would also be a good way of preserving the plant, or freezing the juice in ice cube trays.

Constituents   Flavonoids, including glucosides and quercetin; phenolic acids, including derivatives of coumaric acids; sulphur and potassium.

Planetary influence   Mercury.

Constitution   Temperate.

Actions and indications   Pellitory-of-the-wall is not often used these days, but it yields some valuable medicines for the kidneys, and the urinary tract in general. It is a gentle diuretic and demulcent with an affinity for the bladder, in particular for stones or gravel in the kidneys and any spasmodic complaints of the urinary system. Like many bladder remedies, it is best taken as a tea or decoction. It has anti-inflammatory and gently astringent properties, and so it could potentially be used in remedies for weak bladders or reduced kidney and bladder function, alongside other herbs such as nettle seed, as it supports and maintains good kidney function.

It has been used to relieve some rheumatic complaints, particularly those causing fluid retention around the joints. For the digestive tract, it has been used to relieve constipation.

There is some affinity with the chest and lungs as well, with the herb being used in the past to treat coughs, asthma and related issues, though it is to be avoided during hayfever.

Topically, it can be made into a salve or ointment for piles, varicose veins and gout, or used as a wash or juice to relieve burns and to ease shingles. There is some mention of its analgesic properties when applied to wounds or burns.

Folklore   None really known at present. Pellitory-of-the-wall is another of those herbs that has rather fallen out of favour in recent years, which is rather a shame.

Dose   One tsp, heaped, of fresh herb to a cup of hot water, steeped for 5 minutes and drunk twice a day. Of the cottage tincture, 5 ml (1 tsp) up to twice a day.

Contraindications   In those who suffer from hayfever, pellitory-of-the-wall can sometimes cause hayfever-like symptoms.

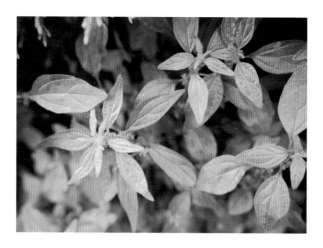

Pellitory-of-the-wall recipes

Pellitory juice for the freezer

Instructions   A very simple recipe, especially if you have a food processor or juice maker. Gather as much fresh pellitory-of-the-wall as you can, roughly chop it, and pile it into the food processor or juicer, then blitz thoroughly, adding a small amount of water if you need to encourage the juices to run properly. Filter the whole lot through a clean muslin and squeeze it thoroughly to express all the juice, then pour it into ice cube trays and freeze it. One ice cube in a glass of water can be drunk up to three times a day to relieve kidney or bladder infection or inflammation. Topically, it can be sprayed onto shingles or burns.

Pellitory balm

Ingredients
- » at least 1 pint of fairly well-packed leaves and stems
- » organic seed oil
- » beeswax

Instructions   This is made in a very similar way to the other healing balms. Simply chop the dry herbs thoroughly and pile them into a double boiler, cover with oil, and simmer for an hour, until the oil turns green. Filter out the herbs, allow 12 g of beeswax per 100 ml (3½ fl oz) of oil, and warm until the wax melts, then pour into jars. Use for bites, wounds, cuts and grazes.

Pellitory-of-the-wall long decoction

Ingredients
- » 2 tbsp, heaped, of chopped pellitory-of-the-wall per cup of water used
- » water

Instructions   This can be fairly time-consuming, but it does yield a much longer-lasting water preparation of the herb. Simply put all the ingredients into a pan on the cooker or wood burner and let it simmer gently for up to 4 hours, topping up every now and then, until the last half-hour, when you are looking to reduce the whole lot down by half. Let the decoction cool, then bottle it. Shorter decoctions can last up to three days in the fridge, whereas this one can last a considerably longer time, though this varies depending on how much the water level has boiled down. Store it in the fridge, and drink 70 ml (2½ fl oz) up to three times a day for bladder, kidney or joint problems. This can also be used as a skin wash, in much the same way as the juice can.

Pineapple weed
Matricaria discoidea

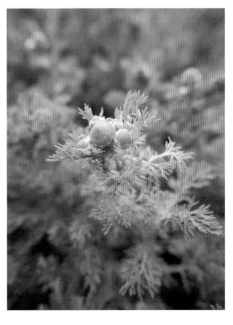

Also known as: false chamomile, wild chamomile, disc mayweed

Family   Asteraceae.

Habitat and description   Pineapple weed is a low-growing, sprawling denizen of turned earth, whether that is because of farm traffic churning it up regularly, repeat digging in the garden, or waste ground in general, particularly in soil that is well packed down, so you will often find it in field entrances and waste grounds in towns and cities as well as among plants growing on verges in country lanes. It has finely divided, pinnate leaves and yellow-centred flowers that have no real petals. The whole plant smells delightfully of pineapple, hence the common name. Like German chamomile, it is an annual.

Where to find it   Naturalised throughout the UK and Europe, pineapple weed can also be found in parts of the USA, particularly the north, and in Canada.

Parts used   Flowering tops.

When to gather   June until August.

Medicines to make   Teas and syrups for calming the nerves; cooling summer drinks; sleep pillows; baths and skin washes.

Constituents   The volatile oil myrcene, and coumarins – there will be many others, but these are the ones that have been researched and confirmed.

Constitution   Warm and neutral.

Actions and indications   As a relative of Roman and German chamomile, it is not surprising that pineapple weed contains some of the same properties. The tea is truly delicious and can be drunk as a calming mid-afternoon beverage to relieve mild

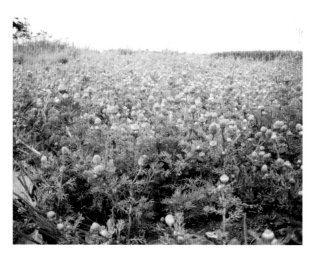

stress and anxiety. It is also very settling to an upset stomach, particularly when this is due to stress. As an extension of this, it is also a gentle antispasmodic and carminative, very useful for the relief of wind, bloating and stomach cramps, as well as for spasmodic period pain.

It is also a diaphoretic and can be drunk hot to relieve fevers and feverish conditions, being a good deal more pleasant to drink than German chamomile, as it makes a much tastier, sweet-tasting tea.

It makes a handy poultice for skin problems, ranging from insect bites and stings to abscesses and boils, and could probably be used as an infused oil for this as well, making it available all year round.

As an insect repellent, it can be rubbed on the temples, or the flowers can be woven into a necklace and worn around the neck. Definitely worth growing in pots on the patio for this purpose if you enjoy eating outdoors in the summer months!

Folklore Pineapple weed was originally introduced into the country in the nineteenth century by Kew Gardens, and promptly escaped, naturalising in the UK over the following years; now it can be found on verges, footpaths and turned earth all around the country.

The Native American peoples used to line their babies' cribs with pineapple weed to deter pests and flies. It has a much longer tradition of usage in the USA than it does in the UK.

Dose One cup of dried or fresh flower heads to a cup of hot water, steeped, sweetened to taste, and drunk up to four times a day.

Contraindications None known at present, though, given its coumarin content, use with caution alongside blood thinners.

Pineapple-weed recipes

Pineapple-weed, limeflower and lemon balm calming elixir

Ingredients
- » one large handful each of pineapple weed, limeflower and lemon balm, fresh if possible
- » brandy
- » plenty of local honey

Instructions   Check over the herbs and chop them thoroughly, then put them into a Kilner jar with four large tablespoonfuls of the honey; pour over the brandy and shake it up thoroughly, then add enough extra brandy to have an extra 2½ cm (1 in.) on top of the herbs. Allow this to steep for a fortnight, then strain out the herbs. Take 5 ml (1 tsp) of the elixir to relieve stress, anxiety and panic attacks – this is a delicious remedy and very effective! It works a treat for stress headaches as well.

Pineapple-weed syrup

Ingredients
- » plenty of fresh pineapple-weed tops
- » enough water to cover the herbs easily
- » sugar to taste

Instructions   Roughly chop the herbs and pile them into a pan, then pour over the water, covering the pan once it has reached a gentle simmer, so that the volatile oils do not escape. Let the whole lot simmer for 10 minutes, then allow to cool, before filtering out the herbs. Allow roughly 500 g (1 lb 1½ oz) of sugar per 500 ml (17½ fl oz) of liquid, returning both ingredients to the hob and simmering gently, stirring regularly until the sugar has dissolved. Bring to a boil for a few minutes, stirring the whole time, then take off the heat and bottle it. This syrup will last up to 6 months in the fridge, and is delicious used to sweeten herbal teas, trickled over ice cream or cakes, or used as a mixer in cocktails.

Pineapple-weed honey

Ingredients
- » 2 handfuls of fresh pineapple-weed plant in flower
- » one jar of local honey

Instructions   Finely chop the herbs and either stir them into the jar full of honey or pile the whole lot into a fresh, slightly larger jar and pour the honey over the top of the herbs. Let them steep for at least a fortnight, and use the whole thing to sweeten teas or just have a small teaspoon to calm anxiety and nerves.

Pineapple-weed butter

Ingredients
- » 1 handful of fresh pineapple-weed flowering tops
- » local honey
- » butter

Instructions   This butter is very simple to make and is a lovely way of capturing that sweet, fragrant flavour. Just finely chop the herbs and, allowing 1 tbsp of honey, mash them into an equal amount of soft butter, until the honey, herbs and butter are well mixed. The butter can be used on fresh bread or pancakes and is very tasty indeed! To store it, wrap it in greaseproof paper and put it in the fridge.

Red clover
Trifolium pratense

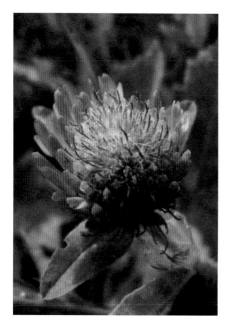

Also known as: *trefoil, purple clover*

Family   Fabaceae.

Habitat and description   A fairly low-growing short-lived perennial that can be found on verges and waysides, meadows, fields and the edges of woodland, red clover contains nitrogen-fixing bacteria in its root nodules, which improve the health of soil. This is a delightful plant to grow in the garden if you can – it can often be found either as seed, or in garden centres that stock wild flowers. Kept in a sunny place, it can be surprisingly long-lasting.

The plentiful flowers are actually many tiny flowers in a small globe, which is fragrant and much loved by bees. The three-lobed leaves have paler green markings on them and are softly furred. You will sometimes find a four-leaved variant on a plant, which in folklore is a very magical thing indeed – if you find them, store them or give them to loved ones. We can all use a little luck these days!

Where to find it   Red clover is native to Europe as well as parts of Africa and Asia but has naturalised in many other temperate regions as well.

Parts used   Flowers, in June only.

When to gather   Late May and June – only the first flowers are used, as the later ones are slightly toxic.

Medicines to make   Tincture, honey, honegar, dried flowers as teas. Dry them in baskets in a single layer, to make sure they do not begin to ferment, preferably in the dark if you want to keep some of the beautiful pink colouring. Tincture or elixir or honegar of fresh flowers, if possible, for balancing hormones and as a lymph tonic.

Constituents   Isoflavones and other flavonoids; coumarins; volatile oils, vitamins and minerals.

Planetary influence   Mercury.

Associated deities and heroes   Freya, Venus / Aphrodite, Hathor.

Festival   Beltane.

Constitution   Cool and moist.

Actions and indications   Red clover has a particular affinity with the lymph glands and nodes, making it a really useful remedy for sore throats with raised glands, for glandular fever or for influenza with raised glands – use it as a tincture or tea for best effect.

It is cooling and moistening and can be used to moisten organs, tissues and joints, especially where dryness is present – this particularly shows up as dry skin, dry joints with a tendency to soreness and a red tongue. It is also gently antispasmodic, so will relieve spasm in dried-out muscles, mucous membranes and blood vessels. It may also be handy in cases of slightly raised blood pressure due to the menopause.

It has also been used to improve nutrition to the brain in cases of overwork and muddled thinking, especially where this presents in getting halfway through a sentence and forgetting what you were saying, or getting easily overwhelmed by details. It can be used to ease anxiety where this is due to dryness and menopausal hormone imbalance. (To those who still subscribe to the Doctrine of Signatures, the shape of the flowers is a pretty good indication for this usage, resembling a little brain at the end of a long stalk.) As a gentle nervine, it can be used for insomnia in children, again in particular where this is due to dryness of the tissues and anxiety.

Use it for long-term constipation where this is due to bowel-wall atrophy and dryness – the mucous membranes of

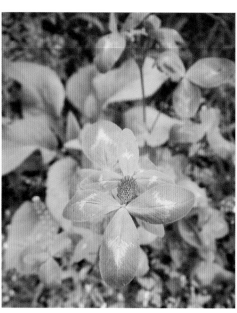

the bowels dry up and make it very difficult to pass a normal motion. It needs to be taken on a daily basis over a long period of time to be effective in this case.

As a superb alterative, it can be used for skin complaints ranging from acne and psoriasis to eczema, abscesses and cysts. Topically, it can be used for this as well – as a skin wash or as a thick poultice made from the thoroughly chopped and mashed fresh plant matter in the case of abscesses and cysts. If you use it for this, also consider herb robert, both internally and externally, to help the abscess heal cleanly afterwards.

The plant is a gentle diuretic and can be used for water retention. Perhaps one of its best-known actions is as a phyto oestrogen, providing extra oestrogen to the body in the case of the menopause and also binding to oestrogen receptors where the body is providing too much oestrogen – in this sort of oestrogen dominance, the body simply has too much of it, which can result in quite a list of nasty side effects, including the muddled thinking, fatigue and tendency to be overwhelmed with emotion already mentioned. Red clover, by binding to the oestrogen receptor sites, stops the stronger oestrogen produced by the body from having so great an effect. If using it for this sort of problem, combine it with some good liver tonics to help the body flush out the excess hormones. I have used it successfully for a variety of issues linked to the menopause, from hot flushes (drink the cold tea when the flushes start to come on) to vaginal dryness and atrophy, and repeat bladder and kidney infections as a result of the atrophy: taken as a tincture alongside herbs such as goldenrod, this can be very helpful. It normalises mucus secretions, so where the body is simply not producing enough mucus, it will encourage it to produce a little more, but, unlike plantain, with its affinity for the lungs, red clover is better suited to the female reproductive tract for this.

Use it both internally and externally, as a poultice for mastitis, as well as for any other issue causing lumpy, sore, inflamed nodules.

Folklore   The four-leafed clover has a long reputation as a handy thing to have to ward off unpleasant or malicious attentions from the faery folk. I used to spend many happy hours scouring the clover fields for them and went through spates of finding several, which I either pressed as they were or dried and stored in little pots. Even as a young teenager I loved odd potions and lotions!

Clover was steeped in the dew gathered on Beltane morning as an aide to beauty and was used to wash the face every day afterwards, until the liquid had gone.

The clover plant has long been associated with the Triple Goddess, perhaps predominantly because of its usually three-lobed leaves, though five-lobed leaves were considered very bad luck after Christianity gained popularity – some schools of thought think that this is because the five-lobed versions were even more strongly associated with the Triple Goddess. The normal three-lobed leaves were linked with Christianity once St Patrick came this way – he used it to convert one of the kings to his faith.

Dose   One tsp, heaped, of the dried herb to a cup of hot water, steeped for 5 minutes and drunk up to four times a day. Of the cottage tincture, 5 ml (1 tsp) up to three times a day.

Contraindications   The coumarin content can convert into dicoumarol, a blood thinner, especially in the older flowers, so use this plant with caution if you are on warfarin or similar drugs. I recommend tracking down a patch of the plant and keeping an eye on it: that way you can make sure you get the very youngest plants.

Red clover recipes

Red clover poultice for mastitis and skin problems

Ingredients
- » at least 1 pint, packed, of fresh clover flowers
- » a small amount of water

Instructions   This poultice is very easy to make and can be frozen for later use. Pack the clover into a food processor with a small amount of water, and blitz it up thoroughly. Alternatively, you can roughly chop the flowers and put them into a large, rough-sided mortar and pestle, then pound them to a thick paste. Pile a heaped tablespoon of the clover onto some muslin or a clean tea towel and apply it to the sore breast, either lying down and using it as some time to rest or, if you absolutely can't make time for resting, use a sticking plaster to fasten it in place. Follow this up with a tea of the fresh flowers, to tackle the problem from both sides. This poultice can also be used for bites, stings, boils and abscesses. To freeze the poultice mix, just pop tablespoonfuls onto a small tray, put it in the freezer, and once the herbs have frozen, pack them into a clean bag or box in the freezer.

To make a skin wash, brew a strong tea using several tablespoonfuls of the herbs in a mug of boiling water. Strain the herbs out once the tea has cooled, and apply using a mister, cotton wool pad or clean cloth. This mix can also be put in the bath.

Menopausal tonic with red clover, dandelion root and sage

Ingredients
- » ½ pint each, loosely packed, of red clover and sage, plus fresh or dried dandelion root, which can be added later if need be, as roots are better gathered in the autumn
- » vodka

Instructions   As with many of the tonics listed so far, just chop the herbs up thoroughly, pack them into a Kilner jar, and pour over plenty of the vodka to cover the herbs. Put the lid on and shake it up daily to make sure the constituents in the herbs extract into the alcohol properly. Leave it for at least a fortnight – if you have added dried dandelion root to this blend, leave it for at least a month, so that it has time to extract properly. After this time, filter out the herbs and take a dropperful three times a day.

Red clover infused oil

Ingredients
- » plenty of red clover flowers
- » organic seed or vegetable oil

Instructions   This oil can be made either on the hob, in the slow cooker, or using the sun method. Simply check the flowers are dry on the surface as well as between each of the tiny pink flowers. Use the chance to look at them very closely – they really are beautiful on much closer observation! Pack the flowers into a clean, dry glass jar, then pour over enough oil to cover them, put a cloth over the top held in place with string or a rubber band, then put the jar in the sunlight. Alternatively, use the double-boiler method, or pile them into the slow cooker with the oil and put it on the lowest setting, leaving it for several hours. This can be used as a breast massage or be added to recipes for healing balms and creams.

Red poppy
Papaver rhoeas

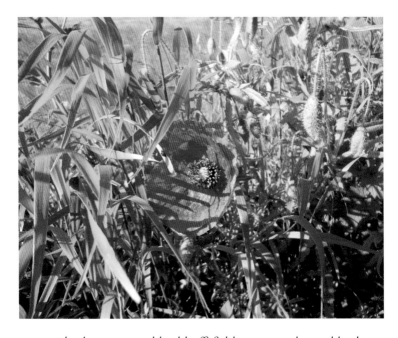

Also known as: blind buff, field poppy, cockrose, blindeyes, headaches, head waak, canker, canker rose, redweed, corn rose, nepenthes, daughter of the field, thunderclap, thunderflower, lightning

Family Papaveraceae.

Habitat and description The field poppy is an annual that tends to grow on disturbed soil, which is, of course, why it is often to be found growing in fields and on road verges. It prefers full sun and well-drained soil. It can grow to around 50 cm (2 ft) tall (less in the fields near my home) and sports the well-known bright-red flowers throughout the summer and autumn. Poppies have lance-shaped leaves with three lobes, which form a rosette at the base of the plant. The flowers are carried jauntily at the tops of tall, hairy stems and are followed by the ubiquitous seed heads, which, when ripe, are pale brown and disperse their seeds readily at the slightest breath of wind.

If you plant red poppies in your garden one year, there is a fairly good chance they will self-seed quite readily, so expect to have them for several years afterwards. The seeds can often lie dormant for years, until the earth is turned enough to permit them to grow. Then they germinate incredibly fast, and so they are most often to be found growing in ground that has been churned up. They were adopted as the national flower of remembrance after the fields of Flanders were covered

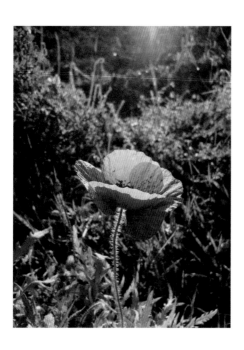

with swathes of red poppies just one season after the terrible battles and losses suffered there.

The field poppy, while related to the ominously beautiful opium poppy, which also grows wild, doesn't contain many of the same constituents, so while it is calming and soothing, it is not addictive or tranquillising.

Where to find it Red poppy is typically a European plant, springing up wherever ground has been disturbed, as was seen after the World Wars. It can be found in parts of Africa and Asia, particularly in the more temperate areas.

Parts used Flower petals, seeds, leaves.

When to gather The flowers can be gathered from June until September, or whenever they finish flowering. The leaves can be gathered from April through the summer.

Medicines to make Poppy petal elixir or syrup or tincture for coughs and sleep; dried leaves as a tea or cottage tincture.

Constituents Alkaloids, including papaverrubines, meconic acid, mecocyanin – the red pigment that provides the poppy flower with its colour and can be used to colour medicines and foods. The plant also contains mucilage and tannins.

Planetary influence Moon.

Associated deities and heroes Hypnos, Demeter, Agni, Ceres, Hades, Jupiter, Harvest Goddesses, Mother Goddesses, Persephone, Pluto, Nyx, Proserpine, Kore, Somnus, Yama, Vulcan. It can most likely be associated with all the assorted Underworld deities to a greater or lesser degree.

Festival Lammas / Lughnasadh.

Constitution Most likely cool and dry for red poppy, but only gently so.

Actions and indications Red poppy is not widely used in herbal medicine. (Opium poppy is really not used much at all these days, because of its heavily narcotic effect, making it highly addictive, as can be seen from the illegal use of morphine.) If used in medicine, the flowers and seeds of the red poppy can be made into a syrup to ease coughs and catarrh and as a mild painkiller, and they are reasonably safe in moderate doses as they do not contain the addictive morphine.

The flower petals can be made into an infusion to soothe the symptoms of bronchitis, catarrh and other respiratory disorders causing pain, as well as the pain of angina. The leaves can be used as a relaxing and soothing antispasmodic for chesty coughs and also soothe the cough reflex for those being driven crazy by winter coughs and colds. They can also soothe digestive spasm and relieve nerve pain such as headaches, neuralgia and shingles – basically, if you are suffering from any kind of spasmodic pain, red poppy may be able to help. I like it best as an elixir, where it can be used on its own or be mixed with a range of other suitable herbs.

I have used the petals in smaller doses to colour wines and syrups attractive shades of rich red.

Lastly, the leaves are astringent and can be used to relieve diarrhoea and to dry up wounds.

Folklore   One old piece of folklore holds that if you soak poppy seeds in wine for fifteen days, then drink the resulting liquid every day for five days while fasting at the same time, you will be able to make yourself invisible at will.

There's a fair deal of folklore associated with the poppy, both the red and opium varieties. The Latin name *Papaver* supposedly derives from *pappa*, meaning breast, possibly referring to the milky sap that seeps from damaged parts of the ripening seed capsule on opium poppies. Alternate legends mention that it was named thus because mothers in the Celtic world would give the sap to fretful children, especially at times of attack in order to keep them quiet and not give away their location.

Greek legends mention that the red poppy was created by Somnus as a way of encouraging Ceres to rest, as she was so exhausted she was neglecting her duties of tending the crops. Ripe wheat and red poppies were the traditional offering to Ceres in the ancient world. According to an alternative version of this legend, poppies were created by the Gods around the feet of Demeter as she rested after spending a long time searching for her daughter, who had been abducted by Hades. The soporific perfume of the plants caused the Goddess to sleep, after which she woke rested and well, ready to continue the hunt. Still another version of the legend has it that the poppies were given to Demeter to make her sleep, as, in her frantic search to regain her daughter, she was letting the natural order of things go astray, and the world was crying out for repose. Once she slept, winter was allowed to arrive, and the land rested. In 1400 BCE, Cretan women worshipped a Poppy Goddess.

The Assyrians called poppies 'Daughters of the Field'. The ancient Egyptians used them in their death rituals to ease the transition between life and death.

In olden times children were warned to be careful when picking the flowers, as it was held that if a petal is disturbed during picking, it can cause storms and lightning. Folklore also speaks of headaches if the flowers are put close to the ear, and blindness resulting from wearing the flowers. Going by all these pieces of folklore, the poppy is a chancy flower indeed!

Dose   One tsp of dried herb to a cup of hot water, drunk three times a day. If using a tincture, I should think no more than about 3 ml (½ tsp) per dose would be sufficient. Of the elixir, 5 ml (1 tsp) three times a day for tickly, irritating coughs works well, or 10 ml (2 tsp) before bed to encourage sleep.

Contraindications   While red poppies do not contain morphine and are therefore not addictive, do be a little cautious using them, especially if you have to drive, as they are sedative.

Red poppy recipes

Red poppy and mullein flower sleep syrup or elixir

Ingredients
- » 1 pint of loosely packed red poppy petals and mullein flowers – equal proportions works best, but use what you have
- » brandy
- » local honey or maple syrup

Instructions   As with previous elixir recipes, make sure your petals are free from uninvited guests – the small black glossy storm bugs love mullein flowers in the summer, so you may have to evict a few of them! If they are a problem, just put the flowers in a basket in a dark corner, and within half an hour most of the bugs will fly off in search of sunshine, making your job much easier. Shred the flowers down and pack them into a jar with the brandy and honey; leave it to steep for a fortnight, shaking it up every other day. Take up to 10 ml (2 tsp) in the evening to give a restful night's sleep. You can also use it in smaller doses – 5 ml (1 tsp) – for tickly, irritating coughs, as well as for panic attacks.

This elixir can be made with just red poppy petals – if you are using this method, just add extra petals as the flowers open. Once you have finished adding petals, let the whole lot infuse for at least another fortnight.

Red poppy leaf tea for simple diarrhoea

This tea is simple to make – just gather a small handful of poppy leaves, chop them finely and infuse them in hot water for 5 minutes, then drink, once cool enough to be comfortable. Be sure, if treating diarrhoea, that this is not serving some useful purpose – removing something from the body that it doesn't want and will make it ill. The last thing you want is to make the diarrhoea turn into something altogether more nasty!

Red poppy, white horehound and plantain cough syrup

Ingredients
- » ½ pint of loosely packed red poppy petals
- » four 25-cm (10-in.) stems of fresh white horehound, or 3 tbsp of dried herb
- » 12–14 good-sized plantain leaves
- » 570 ml (20 fl oz) of water
- » 500 g (1 lb 1½ oz) of sugar
- » 1 organic lemon

Instructions   Thoroughly chop all of the herbs and pile them into a saucepan with the zest and juice of the lemon, then simmer the whole lot for 10 minutes to make a strong decoction. Let the mixture cool slightly, then filter out the herbs through a muslin cloth. Clean out the pan to get rid of any remaining bits of plant matter, then pour the decoction back into the pan with the sugar. Bring to a gentle simmer, stirring regularly until the sugar has dissolved, then turn up the heat until the syrup reaches a rolling boil. Boil it for at least 2 minutes, stirring regularly, then take it off the heat and bottle it.

This syrup can be taken in 1 tbsp (15 ml) doses up to four times a day to soothe a troublesome cough and encourage restful sleep, and is particularly well suited to dry, hoarse coughs where not enough mucus is being produced. It will keep for up to three months in the fridge. Remember to use thoroughly clean bottles, bottle the syrup hot, and, once the lid is in place, turn it upside down to get a good 'seal' on the bottle, which will keep it fresh for longer. Flip-top bottles work well for this purpose.

Rosebay willowherb
Chamerion / Epilobium angustifolium

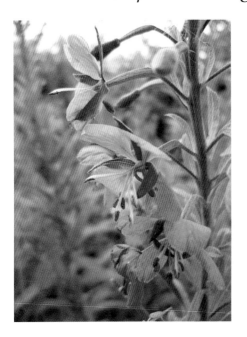

Also known as: *fireweed, thunder flower, London pride, bombweed*

Family   Onagraceae.

Habitat and description   This gorgeous, tall plant of waysides and verges was one considered quite rare in the UK but has since spread merrily around the landscape, mostly via the railway tracks, as it loves disturbed soil. It grows surprisingly tall – up to 1.5m (5 ft) – and has long, oblong leaves shaped like those of the willow tree, hence the name willowherb. The flowers begin to open at the end of July and herald the end of the summer and the onset of the autumn months, providing swathes of bright fuschia and magenta flowers that really are lovely to see, forming in clusters around tall flower spikes. In the autumn months, after the plant has flowered and gone to seed, the whole plant turns stunning shades of copper, russet and yellow, looking from a distance very much like the fire for which it is named, with the open seed pods emitting feathery seeds in charming profusion, looking much like smoke.

Where to find it   UK and Europe, as well as North America, Russia; basically through most of the Northern Hemisphere.

Parts used   The pith can be eaten; leaves and flowering parts for medicine or teas.

When to gather   Gather the pith before the plant is fully in flower. The leaves can be gathered from June through to early September, as can the flowers. The young leaf shoots can be gathered in April and May and eaten much like asparagus. The root is sometimes used as well.

Medicines to make   Teas; infused oils; tinctures; eaten as food.

Constituents   Flavonoids in the leaves; ellagitannins, including oenotherin A & B, which is currently being investigated for anti-cancer properties; quercetin, mucilage and tannins.

Planetary influence   Saturn.

Constitution   Cool and dry.

Actions and indications   Predominantly used as a bladder, urinary tract and prostate remedy, rosebay willowherb – and its cousin, lesser willowherb – is great to have in the store cupboard for relieving cystitis, prostatitis and benign prostatic hyperplasia (BPH). It can be used to relieve BPH because it inhibits 5-alpha-reductase, the enzyme responsible for BPH.

For the digestive system, it is good for diarrhoea caused by relaxed or irritated mucous membranes in the intestines.

By extension, I wouldn't be at all surprised if it was also very handy for constipation caused by relaxed and overheated intestines.

It is considered to be a diffusive tonic astringent with stimulating properties, making it very useful for any ailment caused by over-relaxed mucous membranes. It also has a very useful anti-inflammatory action, probably another of the reasons why it is so good for diarrhoea. For the rest of the digestive system, it can be used to relieve many inflammatory conditions of the stomach and digestive tract, and long-term candidiasis, providing the useful balance of astringency and mucilage.

It also has some affinity for the respiratory tract, making it handy for inflammation of the throat, as well as for asthma and spasmodic coughs.

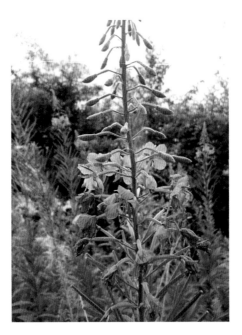

Externally it can be used to relieve eczema, for which it is traditionally used as a salve, though I suspect cool compresses of the cold tea will also be useful for this. Eczema often needs to breathe, so ointments or salves with an oil base can act as too much of a barrier, keeping out oxygen. It can also be used as a salve for arthritis and rheumatism, as well as bruises, bumps and strains.

Folklore   It has a propensity for growing on disturbed ground, which gave rise to the nicknames of bombweed and London pride, since it grew so freely on disturbed ground after bombing raids in World War Two. It gained the name of Singerweed as it grew on the ground left after the Singer sewing-machine factory was destroyed.

Dose   The decoction of the whole herb: 15–30 ml (1–2 tbsp). The tincture dosage is approximately 5 ml (1 tsp) per dose.

Contraindications   None known at present, but be sure that BPH has been correctly diagnosed before using this herb for prostate issues.

Rosebay willowherb recipes

Steamed rosebay tips with garlic butter

Ingredients
- » one handful of the young tops per person, gathered in the early- to mid-spring, before they get too tall
- » butter or vegetable oil
- » fresh garlic, chives, or jack by the hedge

Instructions   Check over the young shoots for any bugs or poop, then steam them lightly for a few minutes. Set aside. Finely dice the garlic and gently cook it in a small lump of butter or tablespoonful of oil until soft, then trickle this mixture over the herbs, tossing to ensure they cover all the plant matter. Serve hot as a side dish or a starter. Alternatively, let it go cold, chop up, and use as an ingredient in spring quiches.

Another method is to cook the butter and garlic, then toss the fresh willowherb shoots in this mixture, letting the heat from the frying pan wilt the herbs. Either method works just fine – experiment and find the one that suits you best!

Rosebay spray for eczema and psoriasis

Ingredients
- » several handfuls of willowherb leaves, plus a couple of handfuls of flowers to give the mixture a pretty colour
- » cider vinegar
- » flower waters – lavender works well

Instructions   Shred the leaves and flowers and pile them into a clean Kilner jar, then pour over the vinegar and let the whole lot sit and steep for a fortnight or longer. Strain out the herbs and add an equal amount of lavender water. If you have any chickweed or cleavers juice left over from spring, add some of this to the mixture as well, to add extra strength to the spray. Pour the whole concoction into a spray mister and use it to douse sunburn, eczema, psoriasis, or to dab onto insect bites and stings.

Rosebay fermented tea

This was often used as a replacement for traditional black tea and is very easy to make. Gather the leaves just as the plant is beginning to flower, and lay them out to wilt for a couple of days. After this, gather up small handfuls and roll them gently but firmly – aiming to lightly bruise or crush the surface of the leaves. Look for a darker, slightly more juicy appearance. Once this is done, the leaves can be left in a warm place to let the flavours mature and strengthen, then dried, either in a low oven or in a dehydrator.

Rosebay tea was drunk traditionally in Russia, and used to be hugely popular in the UK until the East India Trading Company launched a campaign to replace it with black tea. The benefit of rosebay tea over traditional tea is that while it still has a good kick of flavour, it has no caffeine in it, making it more suitable for those who don't cope well with caffeine, and for drinking in the evenings, before bed. Your dried tea leaves can be chopped and stored in airtight jars, ready for infusing as needed. Make your tea up in much the same way as you would black tea.

Rosebay plaister for bruises, bumps, strains and sprains

This can be made one of two ways: either as a basic poultice using the fresh plant, or as the traditional infused oil and salve combination.

The first method simply requires 1–2 large handfuls of the fresh leaves, thoroughly chopped and bashed up in a mortar and pestle to produce a thick, green paste. Pile it onto a large, clean dressing and apply it over the problem area, leaving it in place for a while so the herbs can really get at the bruising.

The second method is as follows:

Ingredients / equipment
- » plenty of fresh leaves and flowers – at least 1 pint, loosely packed
- » organic seed oil
- » beeswax
- » clean tea towel or muslin
- » greaseproof paper, for storage

Instructions   As with most infused oil recipes, check the leaves and flowers are surface dry and clean, then thoroughly chop them and pile them into a double boiler with the oil. Simmer until the oil changes colour, then replace with a fresh lot of leaves to make a double-strength oil. Once this has infused again, strain out the herbs, and allow 15 g of beeswax per 100 ml (3½ fl oz) of oil. The idea here is to make a thicker, heavier ointment that will melt more slowly when used as a plaister. Warm the concoction through until the beeswax has melted. Cut one clean tea towel into quarters, then lay the quarters on a square of greaseproof paper, each on a separate dinner plate. Stir the oil-and-wax blend, then pour it over the squares of cloth, leaving a good 2½ cm (1 in.) around the edges free of ointment. Allow the mixture to set. If you have any spare, either prepare more tea towels, or pour it into a clean jar, so you can use it later. Once the plaisters have set, top with another square of greaseproof paper, roll up, and tie tightly at each end with either cord or a rubber band. Store in clean glass jars labelled with the name, date and use.

To use, unroll a plaister, apply to the damaged area, and bandage in place, firmly enough so the plaister can't slip, but not so tightly that you cut off blood circulation. Smaller plaisters can be made by smearing a layer of the ointment on a clean dressing and simply sticking it in place, but be aware that as the ointment melts, it tends to bleed through the dressing! Leave the plaister in place for at least half an hour for best results.

A lighter mix of the ointment can be used to make a good bruise balm – by just adding 12 g of beeswax per 100 ml of oil instead of 15 g or more. Pour it into jars and allow it to set.

Self heal
Prunella vulgaris

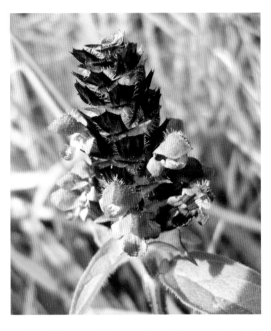

Also known as: all heal, heart of the earth, sicklewort, heal all, hook heal, carpenter's herb

Family Lamiaceae.

Habitat and description This low-growing perennial thrives in scrubland, grasses, meadows, by the side of the road, in the middle of the veg patch – anywhere it can get its little roots in. It is a tenacious but beautiful little survivor, with whorls of leaves growing around the familiar squarish stem of the lamiaceae family. The flowers have the hallmark appearance of this plant family as well and are deep, rich purple, appearing in an almost cylindrical flower head at the top of a stem that rises above the basal set of leaves and has paired sets of leaves growing up it.

My first experience with this plant was in an enchanting story involving a unicorn, where the plant was used to bring the unicorn back to life. Then I grew it, and instead of staying obediently in the herb garden, it decided to grow everywhere: two years later, it was popping up all over the lawn and in the flower beds, much to my family's chagrin. Still, it is a very pretty and useful little plant, so it is better greeted with a smile than a curse. I must admit, this is one of my favourite herbs – it is most certainly one of the first herbs I worked with! These days it fills in the gaps between other herbs and pops up merrily in the grass, providing splashes of gorgeous purple.

Where to find it   UK, Ireland and Europe; North America; parts of Asia.

Parts used   Aerial parts; I tend to gather it when it is in flower; others gather it after it has flowered.

When to gather   July onwards until late August or early September, depending on the weather.

Medicines to make   Infused oils for general purpose healing; teas, tinctures and elixirs for lung and stomach issues.

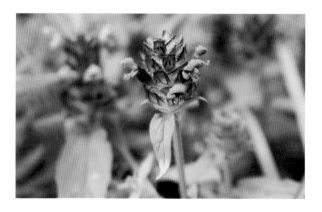

Constituents   Bitters, alkaloids, tannins and volatile oil; flavonoids, including rutin, polysaccharides, and pentacyclic triterpenes such as betulinic, oleanolic and ursolic acids, which are diuretic and antineoplastic; also vitamins A, B, C and K.

Planetary influence   Venus.

Associated deities and heroes   As it has such a long-standing reputation as a healer, I suspect the plant could probably be associated with assorted healing deities – possibly Brighid of the Celtic pantheon, Eir of the Norse pantheon, as well as Aesclepias, Hygeia and the rest of that particular branch of the Greek family of Gods and Goddesses, as these are the ones most usually associated with healing.

Festival   All.

Constitution   Cool and neutral.

Actions and indications   This herb has such a plethora of uses that it really deserves to be a part of every herbal medicine chest. Self heal made into a tea can be used to soothe the discomfort of sore throats, especially when mixed with honey. By extension, it can also be used to ease the irritation of chest infections in general, such as bronchitis. The cold infusion of the herb can be used to soothe hot flushes.

It can be applied as a salve to speed the healing of injuries and, taken internally, to improve healing from surgery and to speed the healing of internal injuries.

The herb is astringent and is also suitable for haemorrhage, for which it can be taken internally and used externally. It can lower fevers, making it a fantastic herb for treating feverish colds and the dreaded influenza, especially where the illness has led to raised glands; it may have some value in treating glandular fever as well. It can be used to return thyroid function to normal, as it is an amphoteric thyroid herb. Self heal can be used to stimulate the immune system and soothe inflammatory responses that cause illness and pain. It can also soothe allergic responses, so it combines well with eyebright, plantain, nettle, ground ivy and mullein in the treatment of hayfever and seasonal-change-related problems.

The herb can be used for the digestive system, to relieve hepatitis, jaundice and simple diarrhoea, and according to some sources, also to improve the body's ability to cope with diabetes by having an action on the pancreas, as well. The flowers in particular are apparently a liver restorative, though I have personally never used the flower tincture on its own.

In addition to all its other useful properties, the herb can be used to lower high blood pressure and resolve oedema, and as a general kidney tonic as well as for haematuria. Because the herb stimulates the immune system and soothes inflammatory responses, it could possibly also be used as part of treatment for fibromyalgia. The antiviral properties also make it handy to combine with medicines such as elderberry and *echinacea*.

Topically, because the plant has such a high mucilage content, it can be used to draw infection out of wounds. A spit poultice can be made of the plant if you are unlucky enough to be out and about when injury occurs, or use a mezzaluna followed by a mortar and pestle to break up the fresh herb.

In China, the herb is used as an anti-cancer treatment, as it has some anti-mutagenic properties, as well as being anti-oxidant.

Folklore   Apparently self heal used to be gathered by the druids in much the same way as vervain. It was to be picked at night during the dark phase of the moon, preferably when the Dog Star was rising, and dug up with the druid's sickle before being held up in the left hand. After this, thanks should be said and the plant separated for drying into flowers, leaves and stems: rather complicated, but, given just how many uses this herb has, perhaps well worth it!

It always surprises me just how little folklore is associated with some of the herbs that have fallen out of favour in modern times. It seems to me that self heal really deserves a far more colourful history than it seems to have at present!

Dose   As with many herbs, no real set dosage is known, so I recommend no more than 10 ml (2 tsp) for a solo dose. For the tea, 1 tsp, heaped, of the herb to a cup of hot water, drunk three or four times a day.

Contraindications   None known.

Self heal recipes

Self heal healing cream

Ingredients
- » at least 2 pints of flowering self heal, picked on a dry day
- » flower water: rose or chamomile both work beautifully for this recipe
- » vegetable glycerine
- » beeswax
- » lavender essential oil
- » organic sweet almond oil

Instructions   For this you will need to first infuse your herbs in sweet almond oil – which was chosen for this recipe because it makes a much lighter cream than sunflower or rapeseed oils. Check over the fresh herbs, picked on a dry day, to make sure they are clean and free from passengers or poop, then chop them as finely as you can using a mezzaluna. Pack them into the top of the double boiler and cover them with the seed oil, then allow them to steep on a gentle heat for at least an hour, until the oil has changed colour. Strain out the herbs and set the oil to one side in a clear glass jug, so that any moisture can sink to the bottom. Once you have poured off the clear oil, it is time for the next step. To each 100 ml of oil you need to add 10 g of beeswax, and then measure into a separate pan an equal amount of flower water to the amount of oil you have used. Add 5 ml (1 tsp) of vegetable glycerine per 100 ml (3½ fl oz) of the aromatic water.

Now, back to the oil mix and the double boiler! Warm the oil until the beeswax has dissolved, then stir it gently and pour it into a clean, dry food processor. Smaller ones work better for this, I find, as you can make smaller batches. While you wait for the oil blend to begin to cool, warm the flower water and glycerine mixture gently, stirring regularly. You are just trying to warm it through, not boil it. Once you can tilt the food processor and the balm still moves, but you cannot see through it any longer, it is time to add the flower waters.

Pop the lid on and add the waters at a gentle trickle, one teaspoon at a time, while simultaneously blending it on a low to medium speed. Use a silicone spatula to scrape down the sides regularly, to make sure you don't end up with large amounts of salve setting around the sides! Keep adding small trickles of the flower water mixture and blending it in until it has all gone and the cream is starting to reach the right consistency. Add 1 ml of vitamin E per 100 ml (3½ fl oz) of cream, plus as much lavender essential oil as you want. (I use approximately 10 drops of oil to 100 ml of cream, simply because healing creams don't need to be strong smelling, just effective.) Blend the essential oil in briefly, then pour the cream into jars before it finishes cooling. Label it carefully.

These pots of cream can last up to six months, but they are not loaded with preservatives, and so they will sometimes go mouldy; if in doubt, store them in the fridge. This cream is great for any number of minor scrapes and bumps, insect bites and stings, and is also wonderful for putting on after the heat has gone out of sunburn. Great for children as well, as the lavender oil is soothing and reassuring.

Self heal, elderflower and elderberry elixir

Ingredients

>   » self heal gathered while in flower – plenty of it. Several large handfuls should do well – I suggest gather until you are bored and dry whatever you don't use for your elixir
>   » elderberries, gathered when fresh
>   » elderflowers, either dried or gathered when fresh
>   » brandy
>   » maple syrup

Instructions   This elixir is definitely a recipe that has to be completed in stages – as is the case with so many of them. These assorted herbs are ready for gathering at different times of the year, so you will need to take this into account when creating your elixir. The elderflower is usually ready first – by around the end of June, though this varies depending on where you live. Gather half a dozen heads of the flowers, strip them from the stems, and drop them into a Kilner jar, pouring over enough brandy to cover them. Put the lid on and put it aside, waiting for the next harvest of herbs.

Self heal is usually ready late June through to late August, and can be gathered when in full bloom. Make sure you get the whole aerial parts – leaves and flowers are all equally important. Finely chop the herbs and pack them into the same jar as the elderflower, stirring it up thoroughly, then pour over some more brandy to cover the new batch of herbs. I tend to add the maple syrup at this point; 4–5 tbsp is usually plenty, but do amend this depending on how sweet you like the remedy to be, and how much brandy you have used.

The last ingredient is the elderberries, which are usually ready from late August onwards. Gather a dozen heads, and strip them off their stems with your fingers. Pop them into a pan with a tiny amount of water and gently warm through, until the berries burst and release the juices. Mash thoroughly, then add this whole lot to the jar, adding yet more brandy to thoroughly cover all of the herbs. Stir up the whole pot and store it for at least another fortnight, to let all the herbs mingle and infuse, shaking or stirring it up daily. At the end of this time, decant the elixir. Take 5 ml (1 tsp) once a day as a prophylactic, or 10 ml (2 tsp) every couple of hours at the first onset of a cold. This elixir will boost the immune system, soothe chest complaints and relieve colds and influenza. It should store in the cupboard for at least a year, but is so tasty that it's a fairly safe bet you will have got through it by the end of the winter!

Self heal cold infusion for hot flushes

This infusion is very easy to make – just gather one large handful of fresh, flowering self heal tops and finely chop them, then pack them into a clean glass jar, pour over plenty of cold water, put the lid on, and put the whole thing in the fridge overnight. This can be drunk cold to ease hot flushes and can also soothe inflamed chest infections, as the cold method of infusing will draw out more of the soothing mucilage content.

Self heal tea for sore throats

Similarly to the cold infusion, gather and finely chop the herbs, but this time put 1–2 tsp, heaped, of fresh herbs or 1 tsp of dried herbs into a teapot or cafetiere, pouring over enough hot water to cover the herbs, then stir in 5 ml (1 tsp) of honey. Let the whole thing steep until it is cool enough to drink as a tea, then strain. Sip slowly, gargling with part of it. If you want to add extra sore-throat tonic benefits, add a little sage to the mixture.

Shepherd's purse
Capsella bursa-pastoris

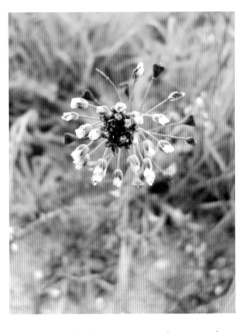

Also known as: shepherd's scrip, lady's purse, witches' pouches, case-weed, mother's heart, pick-purse, sanguinary, pepper and salt

Family Brassicaceae.

Habitat and description This small and easily missed annual and sometimes tender perennial is a denizen of turned and forgotten-about land; it will often settle happily in the vegetable patch, in-between garden plants, and tucked into the edges of field margins and hedgerows where moles have left their mark. It tends to stay small in poor soil but will happily grow somewhat taller in rich ground, with a slender stem rising above a basal rosette of leaves that are quite long and fairly deeply toothed. The flowers are small and white, much like those of bittercress, and turn into charming little heart-shaped seed pods upon pollination, which is one of the plant's main identifying features.

Where to find it   Europe, including the UK and Ireland; North America; China, Japan, Korea and North Africa; parts of the Mediterranean.

Parts used   Aerial parts, gathered for the leaves in spring; flowers and seed pods later in the year.

When to gather   Leaves can be gathered from March until May, and the aerial parts until the end of the summer; best

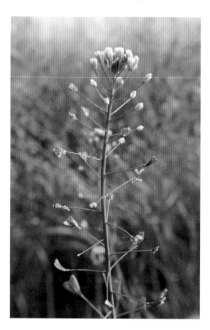

collected in May and June, at the height of flowering and early seed production.

Medicines to make   Tinctures and elixirs for internal bleeding and diarrhoea; salves, creams and wound sprays for external bleeding. The leaves can be eaten as a salad green and are high in vitamin C.

Constituents   Flavonoid glycosides, including quercetin; vitamins A, K and C, and volatile oils; amino acids and carotenoids.

Planetary influence   Saturn.

Associated deities and heroes   Hecate.

Festival   Beltane and Samhain.

Constitution   Moderate and dry. Different folks disagree on whether it is warming or cooling – I personally think it sits pretty much in the middle.

Actions and indications   Traditionally shepherd's purse has a long history of usage for bleeding and haemorrhages, as well as any kind of issues where the body's physical boundaries have been compromised. It was given as a tea or long decoction for all kinds of bleeding, whether from the stomach and lungs, from the uterus, or from the kidneys. It is still used to this day for any kind of uterine haemorrhage, including that caused by the presence of fibroids, and for uterine prolapse. Excessive menstrual bleeding can be resolved rapidly with this herb, especially where this is due to over-relaxation of the uterine wall muscle.

For the treatment of nose bleeds, a strong decoction or the juice of the plant can be used. Soak a cotton wool pad or cotton cloth in the juice or decoction and insert it into the lower part of the nostril. Do this carefully! The last thing you want is a cotton wool pad wadded up and jammed too high up the nose. Leave the cotton wool pad in place for a few minutes, until the bleeding slows and stops. It may also work well as an ingredient in Neti pots for those suffering from regular nose bleeds, as it will act as a tonic to the veins and mucous membranes. Bear in mind though that sometimes nose bleeds are linked to headaches and have nothing at all to do with problematic capillaries in the nose. If you suffer from regular headaches that often turn into nose bleeds, blood pressure is more likely to be an issue, so try herbs like yarrow (*Achillea millefolium*) instead.

The herb also has a strong link with the kidneys and bladder, where it can be used to resolve ulcers and increase urine flow. It is especially useful if mucus is present in urine, or for bloody urine with sand and gravel present in the kidneys or bladder, where it can often bring about a startling cure.

Topically shepherd's purse can be used for all kinds of wounds, including those that ooze and won't stop bleeding, as it has some antibacterial and anti-inflammatory properties that make it a good wound healer.

It has some vasodilator properties, making it of some use for blood pressure issues, though this is usually of short-term help as the benefit is somewhat fleeting.

The herb can be taken over short periods of time to improve internal muscle tone in the case of fibroids, excessive bleeding and uterine weakness in pre-menopause. This use also extends to lax intestine tone, where diarrhoea has become normal, and for digestive systems with lax mucosa where food sits heavily and doesn't digest well or quickly.

As an anti-inflammatory and tonic, it can be of great help when included in healing balms and salves; the bruised fresh herb or salve can be applied topically for rheumatism and arthritis.

The whole plant is edible, but I tend to suggest eating the early spring leaves if possible – I have found that the plants growing locally to me often get rather tough later in the season.

Sources differ widely about the best time to gather this plant, with some saying do not pick it with the white mildew on the leaves that develops later in the season, but others being in some doubt as to whether the plant is as effective if it doesn't have the mildew. For me, I tend to prefer to pick it earlier in the season, before any mildew turns up and before the seed pods go brown.

Folklore   Named for the pretty seed pods, which resemble a commonly carried purse of the time, shepherd's purse only has a limited amount of folklore linked to it. Many of our native small birds love the seeds and will happily stuff their faces with them when they are ripe. The herb was apparently one of the main ingredients in a famous remedy for haemorrhage used by Count Matthei.

An old folk belief reckoned that if you picked shepherd's purse, your mother would die – which is possibly where the old folk name of 'mother's heart' came from, though this may also be linked with the plant's use to stem post-childbirth bleeding.

Use of shepherd's purse goes back a long way – our Neolithic ancestors used it, and seeds have been found in graves dating back to then. Seeds were also found in the stomach of the Tolland man, showing that it has been used as a food for thousands of years. It has also been used for many hundreds of years as a valuable remedy by the Chinese.

Dose   Up to 5 ml (1 tsp) of the cottage tincture up to three times a day, but for short-term use only. For longer-term use in the treatment of kidney issues, go for smaller doses.

Contraindications   Avoid during pregnancy. Large doses can cause palpitations, and, like many of this plant family, it can depress the thyroid, especially if used over long periods of time. This is definitely a medicine, not a tonic.

Shepherd's purse recipes

Shepherd's purse juice and poultice

Ingredients / equipment
- » several handfuls of fresh shepherd's purse: both leaves and aerial parts with the pods and flowers on
- » heavy-duty mortar and pestle
- » chopping board and mezzaluna or sharp knife or scissors

Instructions Finely chop the herbs using the tools you have handy, and pop them into a mortar and pestle one small handful at a time, bashing the herbs up thoroughly before you add the next handful. Take your time – you are aiming to break up the herbs really thoroughly and get the sap flowing. Add a drop of cool water if they are being stubborn. You can put them in a food processor to get them started as well, but, for this herb at least, I tend to prefer to do it by hand, if possible. Once you have pulverised the herbs into a thick pulp, pop them into a muslin cloth and squeeze out as much juice as you can. The green pulp remaining after this can be used as a poultice, while the juice can be frozen in ice cube trays, added to tinctures or healing creams, or used as a skin wash or bath. If you are not going to use the pulp straight away but think you may use it later, just put it into a clean pot and into the freezer, muslin cloth and all.

Shepherd's purse tincture

Ingredients
- » as much shepherd's purse as you need to half-fill a clean glass jar, depending on how much final tincture you would like to make
- » vodka

Instructions   This tincture ideally needs making every year to two years, as shepherd's purse doesn't hold onto its virtues for all that long and usually needs to be made fresh on a semi-regular basis. Check over the plant matter for pests and thoroughly chop it up, then pile it into a jar and pour over enough vodka to cover the plants, plus 3 cm (1¼ in.) on top. Put the lid on and shake it up, then let it sit for a fortnight before straining out the herbs. A good dosage is 5 ml (1 tsp) up to three times a day, though in the case of diarrhoea or excessive bleeding, you may find 5 ml every two hours until the situation is resolved to be a more helpful dose.

Shepherd's purse healing cream

Ingredients
   » 3–4 handfuls of fresh herb
   » organic seed oil
   » vegetable glycerine
   » vitamin E
   » shepherd's purse tea or juice
   » beeswax

Instructions   I make this cream slightly differently to others: instead of flower waters, I use juice from the whole plant, to which I add a tea also made from the plant until I have the quantity required to match the amount of oil produced.

First, finely chop the herbs and infuse them in oil, using a double boiler or bain marie. While that little lot is steeping, follow the recipe for shepherd's purse juice to get as much juice as you can out of the herbs, then use the remaining pulp to make a tea. Once the herbs in oil have turned a rich green colour, you can double-infuse them if you want by straining out the first lot and repeating the process with fresh herbs. Otherwise, strain the oil through a muslin cloth or piece of kitchen roll and return the oil to the pan, allowing 10 g of beeswax per 100 ml (3½ fl oz) of oil. Warm through until the wax has melted, then stir and pour the liquid into a food processor.

While the oil blend cools slightly, measure out the same amount of tea and juice as you have of oil. I tend to do this by putting the juice into the jug first and topping it up with the warm tea – make sure you have allowed it to cool a little before you reach this point. Put the tea, juice and 5 ml (1 tsp) of glycerine per 100 ml of water into a small pan and warm it through until it just starts to steam, then take it off the heat. Once the oil blend has gone opaque but still moves freely, you can start to trickle the water in, blending as you go. Scrape down the sides regularly. Keep repeating the process until all the water and oil has blended together, then add the essential oil you want to use – you don't need to use any if you prefer a non-scented cream. If you use essential oil, blend it again briefly, adding the vitamin E oil as you do. I generally allow 2 ml (½ tsp) per 100-ml jar of cream. Immediately scrape the cream into jars; as soon as the cream sets in the blender, it will become much more difficult to remove, so I advise wiping out the bulk of it with a silicone scraper and following up with a cloth that can be washed easily at a high temperature.

Pop the lid on and label it carefully. This cream can be used for cuts and bruises, sprains and strains, for rheumatic joints and piles, and also for massaging into the breasts, neck and throat to tighten the skin. It will keep for up to six weeks in the fridge – it may sometimes keep longer, depending on the temperature at which you are storing the cream. Remember that creams will separate if the temperature changes too drastically: any liquid that separates off can be removed with a clean cloth or a piece of kitchen roll.

St John's wort
Hypericum perforatum

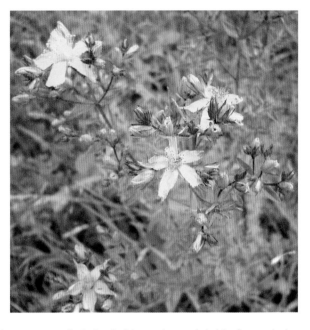

Also known as: holy herb, klamath weed, bible flower, balm of warriors, balm-to-the-warrior's-touch, goat weed, save, herba john, touch and heal, penny john, cammock, tipton weed, amber

Family Hypericaceae.

Habitat and description St John's wort can be grown in pots but thrives best in hedgerows, in plenty of sun, where it grows to up to 1 m (3 ft) tall. Native to Europe, the lovely plant can tolerate some shade but much prefers full sun, growing happily in open woods, grasslands, and on waste ground. The stems are tall and angular, woody at the base and green further up, with small oval leaves that are a delightful tender green colour. Pluck a leaf and hold it up to the sun, and you will see the tiny perforations that the plant is named for: these are oil glands. The leaves grow in opposite pairs along the stem. Between May and September, the five-petalled flowers open; they are a delightful shade of rich gold, in small clusters that open and smile at the sun for a day or two, then wither and fall. The central anthers carry a red pollen that will stain your fingers over time: it is this that lends its colour to the deep red of the infused oil.

Where to find it   Native to Europe, including the UK and Ireland, it can also be found in North America and in most other temperate regions, where it has developed a reputation as rather a thuggish weed.

Parts used   Aerial parts: flowers for a glorious red infused oil, leaves for other problems; the young seed heads can be included in a tincture blend with the remaining flowers and leaves.

When to gather   From June onwards until the end of August.

Medicines to make   Infused oil, salve and cream for skin problems, sciatica and shingles; tincture and elixir for liver issues and for low mood, as well as for its antiviral properties.

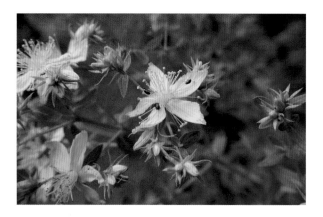

Constituents   Essential oils containing geraniol and limonene, among others; hypericins, including hypericin and pseudohypericin; hyperforin; flavonoids; caffeic acid, and tannins.

Planetary influence   Sun (no surprise there!).

Associated deities and heroes   Sun deities – though the big question is whether or not this applies to all sun deities, or just to the male ones.

Festival   Midsummer.

Constitution   Warm and dry.

Actions and indications   The flowers make a delightful infused oil to relieve inflammatory conditions and act as an antiviral and calming nerve tonic that is great for sciatica and shingles. It can also be used for burns, cuts, grazes and other wounds, as well as for mastitis and tumours, and is a fabulous red colour when sun-infused.

The whole herb has a long-standing reputation in the treatment of mild to moderate depression, for which it is still regularly used in an over-the-counter form. Continuing the theme of the nervous system, the herb is also a wonderful remedy for the nerves in general, for nerve-related pain, spasmodic nerve disorders, and nerve illnesses. It can also be used to relieve anxiety and anxiety-related disorders, combining well with general nervines such as wood betony (*Stachys betonica*) and skullcap (*Scutellaria laterifolia*) for this purpose.

It can also be used to improve the digestive system, being a wonderful tonic for the liver – some caution is advised though, as it is so good at decongesting and improving the health of the liver that it speeds up just how fast the liver metabolises any drugs that your doctor may have prescribed. The CYP 450 chromosome pathway is responsible for metabolising drugs through the liver, and it is this pathway that is potentiated by St John's wort.

As a bitter, it can be used to improve and promote a good appetite and improved digestion, normalising digestive secretions, which, combined with the liver active properties, makes it a great all-round digestive system tonic. Linking together the uses for the digestive tract and mood, it can be beneficial in cases of depression where digestive nerves are affected. Indeed, in many cases of depression or anxiety a close look at gut health is required, in order to rule out the possibility that gut inflammation is causing the problems in the first place, and it may be these sorts of cases responsible for most of the positive comments about St John's wort and depression. Consider combining St John's wort with pre- and probiotics, dietary change as needed, and other herbs such as meadowsweet, plantain and marshmallow, to name but a few.

The whole herb is active against a variety of bacteria and viruses, including *E. coli,* staphylococcus and streptococcus bacteria, as well as AIDS / HIV, Epstein-Barr, herpes, hepatitis C, and influenza; it is a handy one to combine with herbs possessing antibacterial and antiviral properties.

As an anti-inflammatory and painkilling herb, it can also be used for rheumatism and arthritis, as well as fibromyalgia, neuralgia and sciatica.

Folklore   It used to be hung in the window to keep away lightning and also to ward off evil spirits. It was hung in byres and stables to keep away the devil and the evil witches who apparently served him. In mountainous regions of Europe, it was hung in bunches in the eaves and windows to protect the inhabitants and neutralise evil spells. It has been revered for many hundreds of years as a magically protective plant.

Dose   No more than 5 ml (1 tsp) of the tincture per day, or one cup of the herbal tea daily as a tonic.

Contraindications   Can cause sun sensitivity, so avoid sunbathing if you are taking regular doses of St John's wort. Avoid using it alongside time-controlled medication prescribed by your GP – as mentioned earlier, it will speed up the CYP 450 chromosome pathway in the liver, which promotes removal of toxins and medication from the system.

St John's wort recipes

St John's wort flower oil

Ingredients / equipment
- » a plentiful supply of St John's wort flowers
- » sunflower seed oil
- » a double boiler or a large, airtight jar, and a sunny windowsill

Instructions   There are two ways in which you can make a St John's wort flower oil. You can either pack a jar full of fresh, surface-dry flowers, put a piece of muslin on top and place it on a sunny windowsill, or you can pop them into a double boiler and hob infuse them. If enough flowers are added, the oil will, in time, turn a rich blood-red colour. This oil will then keep for some time, and it is a good anti-inflammatory and antispasmodic, good for nerve pain and related issues.

These recipes also lend themselves well to both calendula and meadowsweet flowers. You could also make a rose-petal infused oil, which is very good for the mood and for skin in general. Sun-infusing the petals keeps a lovely fragrance in the oil, which persists for months after bottling and can be used to make beautiful creams and lotions.

St John's wort and calendula healing cream

Ingredients
- » 1 pint each of fresh St John's wort flowers and calendula flowers

» organic seed oil – sunflower or rapeseed works well, as does sweet almond
» beeswax pellets
» vegetable glycerine
» flower water: lavender, rose, chamomile or orange flower works well; to really amplify the healing effects, you can use a good, strong tea of calendula or St John's wort instead
» a few drops of lavender essential oil

Instructions   First, you need to infuse the herbs in the oil. Make sure your flowers are fully dry on the surface and chop them roughly, putting them into the top of a double boiler and covering them with the seed oil. Allow the water in the bottom to simmer and warm the whole lot until the colour of the oil changes – it should go a deep orangey-red colour. Strain out the herbs and bottle the resulting oil. For this recipe, allow 250 ml (8¾ fl oz) of the infused oil and 15 g of beeswax, both of which need to be put back into the top of the double boiler and allowed to warm until the beeswax melts and can be stirred in.

In a separate pan, measure 250 ml of the aromatic water or tea and 10 ml (2 tsp) of vegetable glycerine, and gently warm through. Don't allow the water to boil; just warm it gently until it is roughly blood-heat.

In the meantime, pour the oil and beeswax mixture into a food processor and allow it to cool until it is no longer translucent but still moves freely in the food processor, then put the lid on and turn it on a low speed, trickling in the warm aromatic water very slowly. Stop every few minutes and use a rubber spatula to scrape the oil and beeswax mixture down to make sure it all emulsifies properly; then blitz the whole lot thoroughly once all the water has been added. Lastly, add 5 drops of lavender essential oil to give the cream a gentle fragrance – lavender is very healing in its own right. Use a spatula to scrape the cream out of the blender into clean, dry jars and put the lid on, labelling it carefully. Be aware that this healing cream doesn't contain any preservatives, so it will not last indefinitely, though it should last a good six months. You can use a clean teaspoon to remove a small amount from the jar whenever you need to use some, as a way of avoiding introducing bacteria into the cream. This cream can be used on a whole range of bruises, bumps, strains, sprains, cuts, grazes, insect bites and stings, and minor burns; it is also very effective as an after-sun moisturiser.

St John's wort tincture

Ingredients
- » 2–3 large handfuls of St John's wort stems – gather the top 25½ cm (10 in.) from each plant
- » vodka (buy the strongest you can afford, as it will preserve better)

Instructions   This tincture is very simple to make, especially if you have kitchen scissors or a mezzaluna. Quickly check through the herbs to make sure they are clean and ready for use, then chop them up as finely as you can, packing them into a Kilner jar and pouring over the vodka. Make sure that the herbs are covered by the vodka, with a good 2½ cm (1 in.) extra on top, then put the lid on. Shake up the herbs and the vodka every other day, packing the plant matter back down under the level of the alcohol, and store it out of direct sunlight. After a fortnight has passed, you can filter out the herbs and bottle the resulting tincture. Use it as a gentle mood lifter, a nerve tonic, antiviral and as a potent liver herb: 5 ml (1 tsp) a day is a good dose.

Do not use this alongside medication prescribed by your GP, as it will speed up how fast your liver processes drugs out of your body.

St John's wort, meadowsweet and marshmallow digestive honegar

Ingredients

- » St John's wort flowering tops – go for the top 25½ cm (10 in.) of the plant
- » around a dozen stems of meadowsweet leaves, picked in summer
- » 30–40 marshmallow leaves, or a chunk of the root, which will need to be dug up in the autumn
- » 2 tbsp dried, chopped liquorice root
- » cider vinegar, unpasteurised
- » local honey or maple syrup

Instructions   Thoroughly chop the cleaned and checked-over herbs and pile them into a large jar with the liquorice root, then pour over plenty of the vinegar. I prefer to leave the honey out at this stage, letting the whole lot steep for long enough to be able to ascertain if the liquorice has already made the concoction sweet enough. If you suspect candida overgrowth, you might want to skip any sweeteners altogether.

Let the whole concoction steep for at least a fortnight – I like to leave this one a while longer, because the dried liquorice root in it will need a while to really give its properties up to the vinegar. Once you are happy with the strength of the vinegar, strain out the herbs, and bottle the resulting liquid. Take 15 ml (1 tbsp) in a glass of water per day as a digestive tonic, to encourage healthy digestion and acid balance in the stomach. Please note that this remedy should be used with caution if you are taking any prescribed medication – you should discuss it with your GP!

Toadflax
Linaria vulgaris

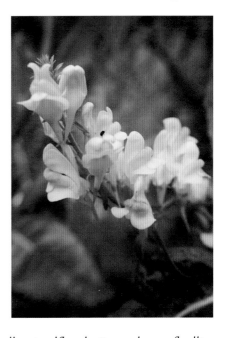

Also known as: yellow toadflax, butter and eggs, fluellin, flaxweed, dragon-bushes, toad, bridesweed, gallwort, pedlar's basket, devils' ribbon, devil's head, bridewort, bunnymouth

Family Scrophulariaceae.

Habitat and description This really rather attractive perennial wayside plant is fairly easy to miss until it flowers, when it has majestic yellow and orange flowers like those of the snapdragon on medium-height flower spikes.

The leaves are fine and palest silvery green, appearing rather feathery; they rise from perennial, creeping roots that allow the plant to spread into large clumps, if given the chance. I find that the plant is quite slow to grow, until mid-summer, when the leaves will suddenly proliferate and the flower spikes appear, at which point it really becomes a bit of a feature plant in the wild garden or hedgerows. The plant likes dry, well-drained soil with a fairly good chalk or sand content in order to really thrive. It has been found growing in crops of flaxseed, which it slightly resembles before it flowers, and where it gets one of its common names from. In parts of the USA it is classed as a noxious weed. Here in Lincolnshire, it is a common sight on untreated grasslands.

Where to find it   Native to Europe, including the UK and Ireland, as well as parts of China, Siberia and Spain. It has also been introduced to parts of North America, where it has since naturalised.

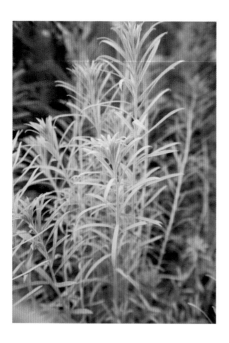

Parts used   Flowering tops and aerial parts.

When to gather   When in flower – July is usually best.

Medicines to make   Infused oil; poultice; dried herb as a tea; cottage tincture; ointments, salves and plaisters for varicose veins or piles.

Constituents   The alkaloid peganine plus choline; flavonoid glycosides, tannin and mucilage. It has rather fallen out of common usage, so has not really been investigated, which is a shame, considering how much our ancestors used and esteemed it.

Constitution   Cool and dry.

Planetary Ruler   Mars, according to some; I, personally, suspect it leans rather more towards Jupiter.

Actions and indications   Toadflax has traditionally been used predominantly for issues relating to the liver and gall bladder and also as a skin cleanser. It is an acrid bitter in flavour and has been used in the past as a warm infusion for liver and gall-bladder spasm or dysfunction, as it decongests the organs, relieves pain and encourages better bile flow. It has been used to dissolve obstructions to the liver and intestines, kidneys and bladder and improves tissue nutrition and blood condition. As a result of this, it is rather useful in the treatment of jaundice, liver obstructions and spleen disorders, and I would be inclined to use it for any ailments or imbalances that stem from this sort of an issue. It can also be used to relieve constipation and haemorrhoids, particularly for cases where constipation is due to a lack of tone of the intestines. Topically the ointment or salve can be used for piles and varicose veins, particularly those with a knotted appearance.

The whole plant is mildly diuretic and well suited to oedema, gravel, cystitis, prostate inflammation and difficult urination, as it contains trace amounts of salts.

It has been used to improve the strength of children with wasting diseases or calcium deficiencies and increases weight and strength, improving health by boosting liver and digestive system function and cleansing the blood, which, in turn, allows the body to gain more useful nutrition from the diet.

Some sources mention that it can be used for sciatica and for those with a tendency to tuberculosis – fortunately not a disease we encounter often any more, but one that used to have a high mortality rate.

It hasn't been much used for quite some time, sadly, but really deserves to be brought back into regular usage.

Folklore   If the chopped leaves are boiled in milk and this milk is then left on the counter, it will kill flies, according to one old piece of lore from Sweden.

Some think the common name of toadflax was given because toads like to shelter among the plant. According to another piece of folklore, the plant was so named because the flowers look rather like toads, with an opening rather like a toad's wide mouth.

One old remedy using the plant was to fry the fresh plant matter in lard until the leaves had gone crisp, which gave a green ointment much used for piles and sores.

An old Scottish superstition held that walking around toadflax three times would break any curse or spell cast upon you; other old folk tales feature toadflax threaded onto linen to protect the bearer from any evil.

The flowers have been used in Germany to make a green or yellow dye, depending on the mordant used with the blooms.

Dose   One tsp, heaped, of dried herb steeped in a cup of hot water; take 30 ml (2 tbsp) three times a day; or 2 ml (½ tsp) of the tincture up to three times a day.

Contraindications   Not suitable for use during pregnancy.

Toadflax recipes

Mugwort and toadflax bitters

Ingredients

- » 1 pint of loosely packed mugwort leaves and toadflax flowering tops
- » vodka
- » citrus peel or coffee or spices or vanilla pod, if preferred

Instructions   Bitters are very easy to make: chop the herbs thoroughly and pack them into a jar, cover with the vodka, and let them steep for two weeks. You can also add flavourings like orange, lemon or lime peel, spices like cinnamon, finely chopped vanilla pods or fresh coffee, if you would like, though it is important to remember that you have to taste bitters in order for them to be effective. Add a pleasant flavour, but don't add any sweetening, in order for the bitters to be at their most effective! You could add a few leaves of wormwood or a bit of gentian or centaury as well if you are feeling brave, but these are very bitter herbs indeed.

Once your bitters have steeped for long enough, strain them and put them into a dropper bottle. Take 5 drops half an hour before meals to stimulate the appetite and aid digestion.

Toadflax and horse chestnut leaf balm for piles and varicose veins

Ingredients

- » flowering tops of toadflax: approximately 1 pint of loosely packed herb
- » organic seed oil
- » an equal amount of horse chestnut leaves, or young conkers
- » beeswax

Instructions   If you are using just leaves and flowers, thoroughly chop the surface-dry plant matter and pile it into a double boiler, covering the herbs with oil and infusing for at least an hour. If you are using conkers, these will need to be bashed up – pile them into a clean cotton bag and bash them thoroughly with a rolling pin – a remarkably therapeutic enterprise! Don't try to do this without bagging them first, however, as they have the habit of ricocheting all over the room if you do. Conkers will need to be infused for much longer – I recommend more like two hours.

Once the herbs have infused in the oil to your satisfaction, strain them and let the oil sit for at least an hour to allow any water to sink to the bottom, then pour off the clean oil. Allow 12 g of beeswax to 100 ml (3½ fl oz) of oil for a simple balm, or, if you want to make plaisters for varicose veins, go for more like 16–18 g of beeswax. Stir over a moderate heat until the oil and wax have melted and mixed properly, then pour salves straight into jars. Plaisters can be poured hot over squares of clean cloth, then wrapped up in greaseproof paper once they have cooled and set.

I have deliberately not added essential oils to this recipe – piles are often better treated with an unfragranced balm. If you are using this recipe to apply to varicose veins and spider veins, then by all means find a suitable essential oil to add, and allow 5 drops per 100 ml of oil.

Toadflax, dandelion leaf, agrimony and corn silk tea for the kidneys and bladder

Ingredients / equipment
- » 1 tbsp each of the dried herbs: toadflax, dandelion leaf, agrimony and corn silk
- » a jar to store your tea blend in

Instructions   Thoroughly mix together the dried herbs and pop them into the jar. Allow one lightly heaped teaspoon of herbs per cup of hot water, piled into a teapot, tea infuser or cafetiere. Pour over one cup of hot water per teaspoon of herbs, and allow the whole lot to steep until the water has cooled to a comfortable drinking temperature. Drink up to three times a day as a kidney and liver tonic.

Recommended reading

For those wanting to continue their explorations into the ancient healing arts of herbalism, here is a list of books that I thoroughly recommend as being enlightening, inspiring and entertaining to read. This is really just a very brief list – there are so many excellent books out there that I haven't yet stumbled across that I have no doubt the list could easily be three times as long!

Alchemical Medicine for the 21st Century – Spagyrics for Detox, Healing and Longevity
Clare Goodrick-Clarke
(Rochester, VT; Healing Arts Press, 2010; ISBN 978–1–59477–931–8)
This is a superb, accessible guide to making your own spagyric tinctures, written in language that is comprehensive yet approachable. If you want to have a go at this elaborate and fascinating procedure, this book will give you an excellent jumping off point.

A Modern Herbal
Mrs M. Grieve
(Surrey: Merchant Books, 1973; ISBN 1–90477–901–8)
This is one of the grandmothers of herb books, and is an immense tome. Worth getting for any herbal historian.

A Woman's Book of Herbs
Elisabeth Brooke
(London: Aeon, 2018; ISBN 978–1–91159–722–3)
Beautifully written and inspiring; particularly well suited to those with a
more feminist mindset.

Complete Earth Medicine Handbook
Susanne Fischer-Rizzi
(New York: Sterling Publishing, 2003; ISBN 1–40270–430–5)
One of the most beautiful herb books I have ever seen – illustrated with
whimsical pencil sketches throughout, and covering some of the more
unusual herbs, with some fascinating recipes.

Hedgerow Medicine
Julie Bruton Seal and Matthew Seal
(Ludlow: Merlin Unwin Books, 2008; ISBN 978–1–87367–499–4)
Covering many of our more common hedgerow herbs and illustrated
with a plethora of beautiful photographs.

Herb Craft – A Guide to the Shamanic and Ritual Use of Herbs
Susan Lavender and Anna Franklin
(Milverton: Capall Bann, 1996; ISBN 1–89830–757–9)
If you are interested in the more magical side of plants, this is the book
for you.

Practical Herbs 1 / Practical Herbs 2
Henriette Kress
(London: Aeon, 2018; ISBN 978–1–91159–757–5 / 978–1–91159–58–2)
Henriette Kress has been an internet staple for many a year now
and was definitely an influence when I was first training. These two
books of hers are superb – approachable and full of useful information.

The Earthwise Herbal – A Complete Guide to Old World Medicinal Plants
Matthew Wood
(Berkeley, CA: North Atlantic Books, 2008; ISBN 978–1–55643–692–5)
Matthew Wood needs no real introduction to any herb lover, and his two
Earthwise Herbal volumes, packed full of information, with more specific
detail for each plant, are worthy of a place on any herbalist's shelf. This

first volume contains entries on a huge array of Old World herbs found in the UK and Europe. The entries are in-depth but somehow still very readable – a good one to curl up with over the winter.

The Earthwise Herbal – A Complete Guide to New World Medicinal Plants
Matthew Wood
(Berkeley, CA: North Atlantic Books, 2009; ISBN 978–1–55643–779–3)
The second *Earthwise Herbal* volume, on New World plants, focuses extensively on American herbs and is well worth having as a companion to the first volume, even if you don't live in the USA – many of the herbs discussed in it can be grown in temperate regions around the world.

The Herbal Medicine Maker's Handbook – A Home Manual
James Green
(Berkeley, CA: Crossing Press, 2002; ISBN 978–0–89594–990–5)
A comprehensive guide to an array of different medicine-making skills, and written in a highly engaging fashion.

The Language of Plants – A Guide to the Doctrine of Signatures
Julia Graves
(Great Barrington, MA: Lindisfarne Books, 2012; ISBN 978–1–58420–098–7)
For those wanting to gain a more thorough understanding of the Doctrine of Signatures and how to use it as a road map, this is an excellent book.

The Medicinal Flora of Britain and Northwestern Europe
Julian Barker
(West Wickham: Winter Press, 2001; ISBN 1–87458–163–0)
Featuring almost all the wild flowers growing throughout the UK and Europe, this is recommended for anyone wanting to gain information on some of the more weird and wonderful of our medicinal plants.

Weeds in the Heart
Nathanial Hughes
(London: Aeon, 2018; ISBN 978–1–91159–748–3)
This is a veritable spellbook of herbs, full of the most stunning illustrations and beautifully written.

Witchcraft Medicine – Healing Arts, Shamanic Practices and Forbidden Plants
Claudia Muller Ebeling, Christian Ratsch and Wolf-Dieter Storl
(Rochester, VT: Inner Traditions, 2003; ISBN 978–0–89281–971–3)
This book takes your mind places. If you would like to better
understand the place of plants for our ancestors, this is a book you may
want to delve into.

Index